Comments on Diabetes — the 'at your fingertips' guide
from readers

'Like a good wine, this book has got better and better over the past 10 years and I will certainly recommend it to my patients, as I have the previous editions. I suppose there must be questions which it does not answer, but it is difficult to think what they are. There is even advice on parachuting and scuba diving which are omitted from many other books. In summary, I think it is brilliant, exactly what one would have expected from the three authors, all of whom I have known for over 20 years.'

Professor Robert Tattersall, Emeritus Professor of Clinical Diabetes,
Queen's Medical Centre, Nottingham

'This book contains just the type of information that patients and their carers really want to know, presented in an interesting and under-standable form. It is this kind of book that gives patients the ability to take control of their lives and run!'

Professor Terry Feest, Professor of Clinical Nephrology
Richard Bright Renal Unit, Southmead Hospital, Bristol

'When I was first diagnosed with type 2 diabetes I read every book I could find on diabetes . . . and then I came across your book in my doctor's surgery. I sat in the reception area when I went for my diabetes induction course and read your whole book in one day – excellent! So well put together and so informative and easy to understand.'

Mrs Clare Mehmet, Stratford

'. . . in style and substance, this is an excellent book. People with and without diabetes will find it very useful. I recommend every diabetic to own a copy of this interesting book.'

Mrs T. Menon, London

'An excellent book. It is comprehensive, informative, and easy to read and understand.'

Don Kendrick, Seaton, Devon

'*Diabetes – the 'at your fingertips' guide* is a marvellous book – just what the layman needs.'

Mrs P. Pilley, Hornchurch

'I like the form it takes (questions and answers); it makes it much easier to find the specific areas when a problem does arise. Also it makes easier reading for picking up and putting down without having to wade through chapter after chapter of heavy medical jargon which for the lay person can be very difficult to take in and understand.'

Mrs Pam Munford, Lincoln

'I have read the book myself from cover to cover and found it to be most informative, up-to-date and presented in a format which is easy to assimilate by the majority of people with diabetes who will undoubtedly relate some question to a particular experience of their own -and find the answer.'

Philip Whitmore, Macclesfield

'I think the book is excellent value since it answers all the basic questions of diabetes and has answers to questions I have not seen written down before. (In fact the whole family is interested in reading it.)'

D. Ball, Nottingham

'My family have found the information in your book of great value – it has been a godsend in many ways – we hope that it will help many more in the same situation.'

Mrs P. Greasley and family, Stoke-on-Trent

'. . . it will be a very useful reference book for patients and health professionals alike.'

Mrs Penny Rodie, Dietitian,
BUPA Roding Hospital, Ilford

'My father has very long-standing and brittle insulin-dependent diabetes who thought he knew all there was to know about his condition. However, he was clearly most impressed with your book and has found it informative and useful. He is a man who is extremely difficult to impress and you have achieved it. Well done!'

Mrs Rachel Booker, Cheltenham

'I have found it extremely helpful and informative, and have learned a lot from it . . . your book is so good and I hope more diabetics will get a copy.'

Mr E R Carr, North Ferriby

Reviews of Diabetes – the 'at your fingertips' guide

'*Diabetes – the 'at your fingertips' guide* is an extensively revised and updated version of the Diabetes Reference Book first published in 1985. The original was an excellent book but this is even better.'

Professor Robert Tattersall, Diabetes in the News

'What sets this book apart from others is the fact that it answers questions that most books dealing with diabetes cannot. It also surprises the reader with questions one perhaps would not even have thought of. Overall this is a most interesting and useful book suitable for people with diabetes, their families, health professionals and anyone interested in diabetes. It is a book that once bought will be used over and over again, and works out to be good value.'

Balance

'*Diabetes – the 'at your fingertips' guide* is a guide, in lively question and answer form, to coping with diabetes. It is quite possible to lead a full life providing the sufferer understands and can control the disease.'

Woman's Journal

'Has positive information to help both young and old lead active lives with the minimum of restrictions.'

Good Housekeeping

'I would recommend it to people living with diabetes, but also to professionals in the diabetes field.'

Professional Nurse

'The book is well presented, with good, clear illustrations and is reasonably priced. I highly recommend it for people newly diagnosed with diabetes and their families and as a source of reference for nurses dealing with diabetes.'

Nursing Standard

'Woe betide any clinicians or nurses whose patients have read this invaluable source of down-to-earth information when they have not.'

The Lancet

Reviews of Diabetes – the 'at your fingertips' guide

'Its strength is that it complements existing texts and is rooted in the practical day-to-day problems and care of people with diabetes. I am sure that it will be immensely useful to general practitioners and practice nurses as well as people with diabetes and their families.'

Dr Colin Waine, former President of the Royal College of General Practitioners

'Its question-and-answer format is easy to read and highly informative. Neither do the authors pull any punches – everything is factual and up to date. Nor is the book only of use to those with diabetes – it would make a very useful addition to General Practice bookshelves and hospital libraries. Look out doctors and nurses who have not perused this edition when confronted by someone who has.'

Diabetes Wellness

'It seems that anything and everything about diabetes in mentioned in this book and the breadth of topics covered is highlighted in the comprehensive index . . . Overall this is a comprehensive, reasonably priced book that would be useful for anyone who lives or works with diabetes.'

Practical Diabetes International

'This text would be of use to health care workers, teachers and people wanting to gain more knowledge about diabetes. It would also be a useful introductory reader for student nurses and I recommend a copy for all nursing and public libraries.'

Journal of Community Nursing

DIABETES

FIFTH EDITION

Peter Sönksen MD, FRCP
*Emeritus Professor of Endocrinology, Guy's, King's
and St Thomas' Hospitals' School of Medicine,
St Thomas' Hospital, London*

Charles Fox BM, FRCP
*Consultant Physician with Special Interest in Diabetes,
Northampton General Hospital*

Sue Judd RGN
*Formerly Specialist Nurse in Diabetes,
St Thomas' Hospital, London*

CLASS PUBLISHING • LONDON

First published 1985; Reprinted 1987
Second Edition, revised and expanded 1991; Reprinted with revisions 1991;
    Reprinted with revisions 1992
Third edition, revised and expanded 1994; Reprinted 1995, 1996;
    Reprinted with revisions 1997
Fourth edition, revised and expanded, 1998; Reprinted with revisions 1999;
    Reprinted with revisions 2001; Reprinted 2002
Fifth edition 2003; Reprinted 2003; Reprinted 2004;
    Reprinted with revisions 2005; Reprinted 2006

The authors and publishers welcome feedback from the users of this book. Please contact the publishers.

Class Publishing, Barb House, Barb Mews, London W6 7PA, UK
Telephone: 020 7371 2119
Fax: 020 7371 2878 [International +4420]
email: post@class.co.uk
Visit our website – www.class.co.uk

Disclaimer: The information presented in this book is accurate and current to the best of the authors' knowledge. The authors and publisher, however, make no guarantee as to, and assume no responsibility for, the correctness, sufficiency or completeness of such information or recommendation. The reader is advised to consult a doctor regarding all aspects of individual health care.

A CIP catalogue for this book is available from the British Library

ISBN 1 85959 087 X

Edited by Michèle Clarke

Indexed by Valerie Elliston

Cartoons by Michelle Smith (ducks) and Christine Syme (foot care)

Line illustrations by David Woodroffe

Typeset by Martin Bristow

Printed and bound in Finland by WS Bookwell, Juva

Contents

Preface to the Fifth Edition

The Diabetes Reference Book first appeared in 1985, was republished with major revisions as *Diabetes at your Fingertips* in 1991 and has been revised and updated regularly since then. The book aims to provide straightforward answers to the questions asked by people with diabetes and those who live with and care for them. The time has come for another extensive revision, for although much remains stable in the field of diabetes care, there have been a number of significant advances in many of the technologies available.

Since the last edition, a large clinical trial carried out in patients with Type 2 diabetes in the UK has reinforced the importance of good control of diabetes and other risk factors such as blood pressure. We want this book to help people improve their health by greater understanding.

Good diabetes care continues to be a team effort between specialist hospital centres, family doctors and practice nurses and a host of other healthcare workers and, of course, they need to keep abreast of improvements in diabetes care. People with diabetes will also want to keep themselves up to date and well-informed and we hope this new edition will be of help to them.

Foreword

by Sir STEVE REDGRAVE CBE

Vice President, Diabetes UK

This book shows a very constructive and positive approach to dealing with diabetes. Its layout encourages readers to develop a good understanding of the condition and to question their approach to the disease. I have no hesitation in commending this book – it helps towards our understanding of diabetes as well as being very constructive in dealing with issues that surround the condition. I have always maintained that 'I have diabetes but it doesn't have me.' Learning more about diabetes is very positive, as is going out and leading a very active and normal life, not allowing diabetes to restrain you in anyway. Happy reading.

Acknowledgements

We are grateful to all the people who helped in the production of past editions of *Diabetes at your fingertips* or the original *Diabetes Reference Book*: Maureen Brewin, Jenny Dyer, Anna Fox, Professor Harry Keen, Julia Kidd, Lis Lawrence, Gary Mabbutt, Pat McDowell, Sheila Nicholass, Sara Moore, the late Sir Harry Secombe, Michelle Smith, and Peter Swift.

We should also like to thank the following people for their contributions to the third edition:

Gill Jowett for revising the section on feet;

Clara Lowy for contributing to the chapter on pregnancy;

Jill Metcalfe for the section on diet;

Suzanne Lucas at Diabetes UK for valuable comments;

Judith North and Janet Waterson for very helpful and practical suggestions;

Christine Syme for the cartoons on foot care.

In the fourth edition, Dawn Kenwright gave us valuable advice about running, and Prue Richardson made a major contribution.

In this fifth edition the Care Department of Diabetes UK made very valuable comments, as well as supplying us with fact sheets and giving us website references for information we lacked. Sara Moore, Isabelle Drayton, Clare Lemon and Norma McGough gave invaluable practical advice, for which we are very grateful. Acknowledgements are due to Derrick Cutting for Table 2.1, taken from his book *Stop that heart attack!*, published by Class

Publishing, and to Susie Orbach for her advice on diet for babies and children in the box in Chapter 8.

We thank the companies who kindly provided illustrations:

Aventis Pharma
Bayer
BD Diabetes Health Care
Lifescan
Novo Nordisk Pharmaceuticals

We thank also the long-suffering patients at St Thomas' Hospital and Northampton General Hospital. They have asked many of the questions and have worked out solutions to most of the problems. We are simply passing on their experience to others. Finally, many thanks to all those who have written in for advice. Some of their questions have been incorporated.

Peter Sönksen
Charles Fox
Sue Judd

Note to reader

There is a glossary at the end of this book to help you with any words that may be unfamiliar to you. If you are looking for particular topics, you can use either the detailed list of Contents on pp. vii–x or the Index, which starts on p. 305.

Introduction

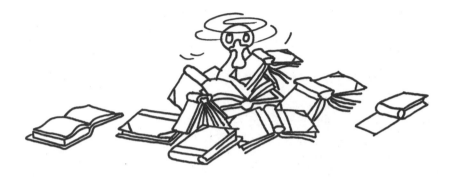

When diabetes suddenly hits you or a close relative, many unpleasant things come to mind, such as injections, strict diets, urine tests, blindness. In fact most people with diabetes do not need injections, their diet is normal and wholesome, urine tests have gone out of fashion and eye disease can now be successfully treated. However, people do have to learn to control their diabetes and they can do this only by understanding the condition. Much advice and help comes from nurses, doctors, dietitians and others, but how well the condition is controlled is each individual's own decision. A lot of effort is being put into diabetes education and this book is part of that effort. There is a great deal of information for all of us to learn.

Diabetes is a complex disorder, and parts of this book reflect its complexity. Although some aspects of diabetes are hard to understand, most people manage to lead full lives by incorporating their condition into their normal work and activities. If you have just discovered that you (or a close relative) have diabetes, you will probably feel shocked and worried. This is not the time to try to learn about the most difficult aspects of the subject. But even at this early stage you, your partner, and your parents if you are a child, need to know certain basic facts. Once the initial shock reaction is over and your own experience with diabetes increases, you will be ready to learn about the frills. Remember that no one involved in this subject (including doctors and nurses) ever stops learning more about it.

How to use this book

This book is a series of questions and answers, and it is not designed to be read from cover to cover. Some of the sections do stand on their own, in particular those describing the nature of diabetes in Chapter 1, Chapter 4 on control of diabetes and Chapter 9 on long-term complications.

If you are newly diagnosed, you may not be ready to come to grips with Chapter 10 on research but you may want to find out about what is known about the causes of diabetes (in Chapter 1). If you have just started insulin injections you should read the following sections at an early stage:

- Hypos (in Chapter 3)
- Other illnesses (in Chapter 5)
- Insulin (in Chapter 3)
- Control and monitoring (in Chapter 4)
- Blood glucose (in Chapter 4)
- Driving (in Chapter 5)
- Emergencies (in Chapter 12)

More experienced people will want to test us out in our answers in Chapter 5 on life with diabetes to see if our answers coincide with their own experience. Parents of children with diabetes will want to read Chapter 8 on diabetes in the young.

There is bound to be some repetition in a book of this sort, but we think it is better to deal with similar topics under separate headings rather than ask the reader to shuffle from one end of the book to the other. We hope that at least we are consistent in our answers.

Feedback is the most important feature of good diabetes care. This relies on people being honest with the doctor or nurse and vice versa. Not everyone will agree with the answers we give, but the book can only be improved if you let us know when you disagree and have found our advice to be unhelpful. We would also like to know if there are important questions that we have not covered. Please write to us c/o Class Publishing, Barb House, Barb Mews, London W6 7PA, UK.

1
All about diabetes

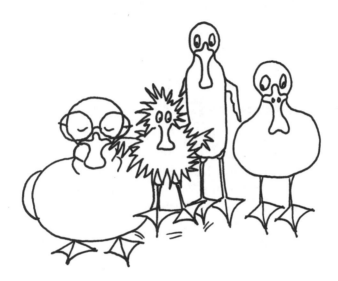

This chapter opens with a description of the central problem in diabetes, which is an increase in the amount of glucose (sugar) in the blood. We describe why this happens and why it may be dangerous. There are two main types of people with diabetes:

- Type 1 – this type of diabetes usually appears in younger people under the age of 40. It is treated by insulin injections and diet;
- Type 2 – this type of diabetes usually appears in people over the age of 40. They may have had undetected diabetes for many years and may not feel particularly unwell. Diabetes in older people is often discovered by chance and commonly responds well to diet or tablets, although in due course insulin and dict may be needed.

There are other rare types of diabetes, which we also mention in this chapter.

Someone with diabetes might feel before the condition is diagnosed and treated. Once treatment has been started, people with diabetes should feel perfectly well. We also make the point that older people may have diabetes and yet feel quite well in themselves. In such cases the condition will be discovered following a routine blood or urine test for glucose, and diabetes may therefore exist for many years without being discovered. Unfortunately undetected diabetes over a period of years may lead to complications affecting eyes, nerves and blood vessels.

What is diabetes?

The pancreas is a gland situated in the upper part of your abdomen and connected by a fine tube to your intestine (see Figure 1.1). One of its functions is to release digestive juices, which are mixed with food soon after it leaves your stomach.

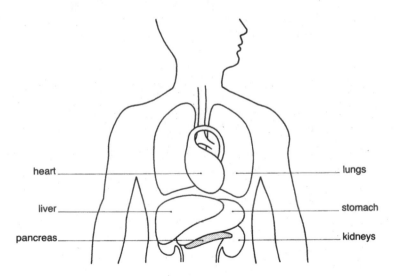

Figure 1.1 Location of the pancreas

These are needed for digestion and absorption of food into your body. This part of the pancreas has nothing to do with diabetes.

Your pancreas also produces a number of hormones, which are released directly into your bloodstream, unlike the digestive juices which pass into the intestine. The most important of these hormones is insulin, the shortage of which causes diabetes. The other important hormone produced by the pancreas is glucagon, which has the opposite action to insulin and may be used in correcting serious hypos (see the section on *Hypos* in Chapter 3 for more information about this). Both hormones come from a part of your pancreas known as the islets of Langerhans.

Why does my body need insulin?

Without insulin the body cannot make full use of food that is eaten. Normally, food is eaten, taken into the body and broken down into simple chemicals, such as glucose, which provide fuel for all the activities of the body. These simple chemicals also provide building blocks for growth or replacing worn-out parts, and any extra is stored for later use. In diabetes, food is broken down as normal but, because of the shortage of insulin or because insulin does not work properly, excess glucose is not stored and builds up in the bloodstream, spilling over into the urine. Insulin ensures that a perfect balance is kept between the production of glucose by the liver and its use.

The breakdown of food takes place in the liver, which can be regarded as a food processing factory. Glucose is one of the simple chemicals made in the liver from all carbohydrate foods. In the absence of insulin, glucose pours out of the liver into the bloodstream. Insulin switches off this outpouring of glucose from the liver and causes glucose to be stored in the liver as starch or glycogen. Insulin also helps glucose to get into cells where it is used as a fuel. Insulin has a similar regulatory effect on amino acids and fatty acids, which are the breakdown products of protein and fat respectively.

What happens to the insulin production in diabetes?

In people without diabetes, insulin is stored in the pancreas and released into the blood as soon as the blood glucose level starts to rise after eating. Insulin is released straight into the liver where it has the important role of regulating glucose production and promoting the storage of glucose as glycogen. The level of glucose in the blood then falls and, as it does so, insulin production is switched off (see Figure 1.2). Thus people who do not have diabetes have a very sensitive system for keeping the amount of glucose in the blood at a steady level.

In diabetes this system is faulty. People with Type 2 diabetes can still produce some insulin but not in adequate amounts to keep the blood glucose level normal. This is because their insulin does not work properly (a condition called 'insulin resistance'). People with Type 1 diabetes have little or no insulin of their own and need injections of insulin to try to keep the blood glucose level normal. Even if given four or five times a day, an injection of insulin is not as efficient at regulating blood glucose as the pancreas, which responds to small changes in blood glucose by switching the insulin supply on or off at a moment's notice.

There are three main factors affecting your blood glucose:

- food (which puts it up)
- insulin
- exercise (which both bring it down).

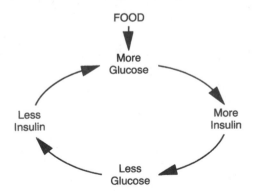

Figure 1.2 Insulin production system

Any form of stress, in particular an illness like 'flu, puts up your blood glucose. Learning how to balance your blood glucose level is a matter of trial and error. This involves taking a lot of measurements and discovering how various foods and forms of exercise affect your blood glucose.

In the past, people with Type 1 diabetes were brought into hospital to be 'stabilized' on a certain dose of insulin. Experience has shown that the insulin needed in the artificial surroundings of a hospital ward bears little relation to the amount needed in someone leading an active life in the outside world. Nowadays, you can 'stabilize' your own diabetes at home yourself. You will find information to help you do this in Chapter 3 on *Treatment with insulin* and Chapter 4 on *Monitoring and control*.

Types of diabetes

I hadn't realised that there were different types of diabetes until was diagnosed with what my GP called Type 2. What is the difference between my diabetes and Type 1 diabetes?

Diabetes does exist in many different forms. Two main groups are recognized:

- Type 1 diabetes is found in younger people under 40 years old. This condition develops in a dramatic way and insulin injections are nearly always needed. About 1 in 10 of all people with diabetes fall into this category, which used to be called insulin dependent diabetes.
- At the other end of the scale Type 2 diabetes occurs in older people, who often are overweight, and have less obvious symptoms. Obesity is linked to insulin resistance, which is a root cause of Type 2 diabetes. Insulin resistance occurs many years before diabetes itself begins. At the onset of Type 2 diabetes, treatment is with diet with or without tablets. After a few years, people with Type 2 diabetes may need to use insulin.

There are plenty of exceptions to this rule. Occasionally young people can be well controlled with diet or tablets and a large number of people who develop diabetes late in life are much better off on insulin injections.

I have been told that I have diabetes insipidus? Is this the same as the diabetes that my friend's elderly father has?

The only connection between *diabetes insipidus* and the more common form of diabetes (where the full name is *diabetes mellitus*) is that people with both conditions pass large amounts of urine. Diabetes insipidus is a rare condition caused by an abnormality in the pituitary gland and not the pancreas. One disorder does not lead to the other, and diabetes insipidus does not carry the risk of long-term complications found in diabetes mellitus.

My wife has just given birth to a baby boy who weighed 4.3 kg (9 lb) at birth. Apparently she may have had diabetes while she was pregnant. Is this likely to happen again with her next baby?

Women who give birth to heavy babies (over 4 kg or 9 lb) may have had a raised blood glucose level during pregnancy. This extra glucose crosses into the unborn baby, who responds by producing extra insulin of its own. The combination of excess glucose and excess insulin makes the unborn baby grow fat and bloated. After birth the baby is cut off from the high glucose input and then runs the risk of a low glucose concentration (*hypoglycaemia*). Overweight babies of mothers with diabetes are at risk of hypoglycaemia.

Women who develop diabetes during pregnancy and return to normal after delivery have a condition called *gestational diabetes*. Once the problem has been identified, it is very likely to recur during subsequent pregnancies. Provided that glucose levels are kept within normal limits (insulin may be needed for this), the baby will be a normal weight and will not be at risk.

Women who have diabetes during pregnancy are more likely to develop diabetes later in life.

Causes of diabetes

Despite a vast amount of research throughout the world the cause of diabetes is not known. Some families carry an extra risk of diabetes (see the next section on *Inheritance*) and the disease may follow an infection such as a cold.

Why have I got diabetes?

The short answer is that your pancreas is no longer making enough insulin for your body's needs. The long answer as to why this has happened to you is not so well understood but there are a few clues. Diabetes often runs in families (see the next section on *Inheritance*). Other possible causes are discussed in this section. It is not a rare condition and in the UK, about 3 people in 100 are known to have diabetes, with an equal number of people who have diabetes but are unaware of it. If a whole population is carefully screened for diabetes, many new people with diabetes are discovered, usually 1 new one for every known one. About 3 children per 1000 have diabetes and the risk is increasing, particularly in young children below the age of 5 years.

Could diabetes be triggered by a virus?

Some scientists used to suspect that a certain virus could be the cause of diabetes in young people but proof is lacking and this theory now seems very unlikely.

There is certainly no 'diabetes virus' and you cannot catch diabetes like chickenpox. There is no suggestion that diabetes in older people could be caused by a virus infection.

I was very overweight when I was diagnosed with diabetes. Can this have caused my diabetes?

If the tendency or genetic makeup towards diabetes is present, then being obese (or even just overweight) may bring on the disease. This is because being overweight, particularly carrying excess fat around the abdomen (central obesity), stops insulin from lowering blood sugar properly (called insulin resistance). This is the common cause of diabetes in middle-aged or older people and is generally rare in young people. However, in parts of the western world where young people are often very obese, Type 2 diabetes is becoming common in children. In most cases this type of diabetes can be controlled at first by dieting and weight loss. Many people with diabetes who are overweight find it hard to lose weight; others find that strict dieting alone is insufficient to lower the blood glucose and have to take tablets or have insulin injections. This is second best, as the sensible and safe treatment for an overweight older person is weight loss.

You will find more information about diet and diabetes and being overweight in Chapter 2.

Is diabetes a disease of modern times?

The earliest detailed description of diabetes was made 2000 years ago but it is much more common now than in the past. This is particularly true of Type 2 diabetes, which is becoming very common in some countries such as India. Diabetes in younger people is also becoming more common, and this has been related to increasing affluence and obesity.

My mother died very suddenly last year and not long afterwards I was diagnosed with diabetes. Can a bad shock bring on diabetes?

Sometimes diabetes develops soon after a major disturbance in life, such as a bereavement, a heart attack or a bad accident, and the diabetes is blamed on the upset. This is not really the case, as insulin failure in the pancreas takes a long time to develop. However, a bad shock could stress your system and bring on diabetes a bit earlier if your insulin supply is already running low.

I was very ill last year and developed diabetes, which has since got better. Can a severe illness cause diabetes?

Any serious medical condition (such as a heart attack or injuries from a traffic accident) can lead to diabetes. This is because the hormones produced in response to stress tend to oppose the effect to insulin and cause the glucose level in the blood to rise. Most people simply produce more insulin to keep the blood glucose stable. However, in some cases, if the reserves of insulin are inadequate, the blood glucose level will climb. You had temporary diabetes, and the glucose level returned to normal once your stress was over. However, you will carry an increased risk of developing permanent diabetes later in life.

My latest baby was very big at birth. Would she have caused me to have developed diabetes?

No, the opposite is true. In any woman who has given birth to a baby weighing more than 4 kg (9 lb), the possibility of diabetes should be considered by her doctors or midwives. If you had diabetes during pregnancy but recovered soon after your baby was born, you will carry an increased risk of diabetes for the rest of your life. The baby itself does not carry this risk.

Diabetes and pregnancy are dealt with in detail in Chapter 7.

Was there anything I should have done to prevent my diabetes?

No. At the present time, if you are going to get diabetes, you get diabetes. It is possible, under certain circumstances, to identify some people who do not have diabetes but who have a very high risk of developing it in the future. Various drugs have been tried to prevent diabetes in these high-risk people, but so far with no lasting success. In the case of Type 2 diabetes, a strict programme of exercise and weight loss has been shown to delay delay the onset of diabetes.

My doctor said that the drugs I am taking for asthma might have caused my diabetes. Is this true?

Yes, several drugs in common use can either precipitate diabetes as an unwanted side effect or make existing diabetes worse. The most important group of such medicines are hormones.

Hormones are substances produced by special glands in the body and insulin from the pancreas is an example of a hormone. Some hormones have an anti-insulin effect and one of these, a steroid hormone, is often used to treat such medical conditions as severe asthma or rheumatoid arthritis. The most commonly used steroid is prednisolone, which opposes insulin and therefore puts up the level of glucose in the blood. Steroids in large doses will often precipitate diabetes, which usually gets better when the steroids are stopped.

The contraceptive pill is another type of steroid hormone with a mild anti-insulin effect. Sometimes people on insulin find that they have to give themselves more insulin while taking the pill.

Glucagon is a hormone from the pancreas with a strong anti-insulin effect. It is used to correct a severe insulin reaction (see the section on **Hypos** in Chapter 3 for how and when to use glucagon).

Apart from other hormones, certain medicines, such as water tablets (diuretics) may have an anti-insulin effect and precipitate diabetes.

I have recently been given steroid treatment (prednisolone) for severe arthritis. My joints are better but my doctor has now found sugar in my urine and tells me I have diabetes. Is this likely to be permanent?

Steroids are effective treatment for a number of conditions but they may cause side effects, as you have just discovered. One of these is to cause diabetes, which can sometimes be controlled with tablets (e.g. gliclazide). However if large doses of steroids are being used, people often need insulin to control the blood glucose. When you stop steroid therapy, there is a good chance that the diabetes will go away completely.

However, you may have had diabetes without knowing it before you started on steroids, in which case you will continue to have diabetes after stopping steroids and will need to continue some form of treatment indefinitely.

I am told that other hormones that the body produces, apart from insulin, may cause diabetes. Is this true?

It is a deficiency of enough insulin to meet demand that leads to diabetes. Sometimes excessive amounts of other hormones will tend to push the blood sugar levels up. If the body cannot respond with enough extra insulin, diabetes may result. Thus someone who produces too much thyroid hormone ('thyrotoxicosis' or 'hyperthyroidism') may develop diabetes, which clears up when their thyroid is restored to normal. Thyrotoxicosis and diabetes tend to run together in families, and people with one of these conditions are more likely to develop the other.

Sometimes a person will produce excessive quantities of steroid hormones (*Cushing's disease* or Cushing's syndrome), and this may lead to diabetes (see the previous two questions for the connection between steroids and diabetes). *Acromegaly* is a condition where excess quantities of growth hormone are produced and this too may lead to diabetes.

I have had to go to hospital for repeated attacks of pancreatitis and now have diabetes. I am told that these two conditions are related – is this true?

Pancreatitis means that your pancreas has become inflamed and this can be a very painful and unpleasant illness. The pancreas is the gland that produces insulin as well as other hormones and digestive juices. If it is severely inflamed or damaged, it may not be able to produce enough insulin. Sometimes diabetes develops during or after an attack of pancreatitis and tablets or insulin are needed to keep control of the blood glucose. This form of diabetes is usually, but not always, permanent.

What other diseases would increase the chances of getting diabetes?

There are four groups of such diseases:

- **Glandular disorders**, in particular thyrotoxicosis (overactive thyroid), acromegaly (excess growth hormone) and Cushing's disease (excess steroid hormone) (see an earlier question).
- **Diseases of the pancreas**, including pancreatitis, cancer of the pancreas, iron overload (haemochromatosis) and cystic fibrosis (a serious inherited childhood disorder); surgical removal of the pancreas (for either pancreatitis or cancer) also causes diabetes.
- **Virus diseases**, such as rubella (German measles), mumps and Coxsackie virus can be very rare causes of diabetes.
- **Medical problems**, such as heart attacks, pneumonia and major surgical operations put stress on the body; the diabetes usually clears up when the stress is removed but these individuals may be more at risk of diabetes.

You will find more information about the relationships between these disorders and diabetes in other questions earlier in this chapter.

Symptoms

Why does someone of my son's age (he is 11) feel thirsty when diabetes is first discovered?

The first signs of diabetes in a young person are thirst and loss of weight. These two symptoms are related and one leads to the other (we deal in more detail with weight loss in the answer to the next question). The first thing to go wrong is the increased amount of urine. Normally we pass about 1½ litres (approximately 2 pints) of urine per day but people with uncontrolled diabetes may produce five times that amount. The continual loss of fluid dries out the body and the sensation of thirst is a warning that, unless they drink enough to replace the extra urine, they will soon be in trouble.

Of course people who do not have diabetes may also pass large amounts of urine. Every beer drinker knows the effects of 5 pints of best bitter! In this case the beer causes the extra urine, whereas in diabetes the extra urine causes the thirst. In the early stages, the resulting thirst is usually mild and most people fail to realize its significance unless they have had some personal experience of diabetes. Someone with undiagnosed diabetes may take jugs of water up to bed, wake in the night to quench their thirst and pass urine, and still not realize that something is wrong. It would be helpful if more people knew that unexplained thirst may be due to diabetes.

I had lost quite a lot of weight before I was finally diagnosed with diabetes. Why was this?

The main fuel for the body is glucose, which is obtained from the digestion of sugary or starchy food. People with untreated diabetes have too much glucose in their bloodstream and this glucose overflows into the urine and also cannot properly use the sugar to provide energy and build tissues. Body tissues are broken down to form glucose and ketones (see the section on *Urine testing* in Chapter 4), and this causes weight loss.

Someone who has uncontrolled diabetes may lose as much as 1000 g (just over 2 lb) of glucose (sugar) in their urine in 24 hours. Anyone trying to lose weight knows that sugar = calories. These calories contained in the urine are lost to the body and are a drain on its resources. The 1000 g of glucose lost are equivalent to 20 currant buns (4000 calories per day).

My vagina has been really itchy and sore. My GP says it's to do with my diabetes. Can this be right?

A woman whose diabetes is out of control may be troubled by itching around her vagina. The technical name for this distressing symptom is *pruritus vulvae*. The equivalent complaint may be seen in men when the end of the penis becomes sore (*balanitis*). If the foreskin is also affected, it may become thickened (*phimosis*), which prevents the foreskin from being pulled back and makes it difficult to keep the penis clean.

These problems are the result of infection from certain yeasts, which thrive on the high concentration of glucose in this region. If you keep your urine free from glucose by good control of your diabetes, the itching and soreness will normally clear up. Anti-yeast cream from your doctor may speed up the improvement but this is only a holding measure while glucose is cleared from your urine.

I have had blurred vision for a weeks now. Can my eyesight be affected early on in diabetes?

The lens of the eye is responsible for focusing the image on the retina. Blurred vision is usually a temporary change, which can be corrected by wearing glasses. The lens of the eye becomes swollen when diabetes is out of control and this leads to short-sightedness. As the diabetes comes under control, so the lens of the eye returns to normal. A pair of glasses fitted for a swollen lens at a time of uncontrolled diabetes will no longer be suitable when the diabetes is brought under control. If you have been newly diagnosed with diabetes and find that you have blurred vision, you should wait for a few months after things have settled down before visiting an optician for new spectacles. The blurred vision may improve on its own and new glasses may not be needed.

Most of the serious eye problems caused by diabetes are due to damage to the retina (*retinopathy*). The retina is the 'photographic plate' at the back of the eye. Even minor changes in the retina take several years to develop but older people may have diabetes for years without being aware of it. In such cases the retina may already be damaged by the time diabetes is diagnosed.

In very rare cases the lens of the eye may be permanently damaged (*cataract*) when diabetes is badly out of control.

You will find more information about the effect of diabetes on the eyes in the section on *Eyes* in Chapter 9.

Can diabetes be discovered by chance?

Yes, but this usually happens only in Type 2 diabetes. In Type 1 diabetes the diagnosis is usually made because someone feels unwell and goes to the doctor.

In older people with no obvious medical problems, diabetes is often discovered as a result of a routine urine test – say in the course of an insurance examination. Once the diagnosis is made, the person may admit to feeling slightly thirsty or tired, but these symptoms may not be very dramatic, and are often put down to 'old age'. So, in older people, diabetes may appear to be a minor problem, but must be taken very seriously as so-called 'mild' diabetes can lead to serious problems. In any case, people often feel better with more energy once diabetes is controlled, often by diet or by diet and tablets, although in the long run insulin injections may be needed.

I have been told that I have 'fatty liver'. Did my diabetes cause this and is there anything one can do to help reverse the situation?

Your liver may become enlarged in cases of poorly controlled diabetes, owing to an accumulation of fat within the substance of the liver. Insulin plays an important part in the metabolism of fat and, when the insulin supply is deficient, the levels in the blood of both glucose and fat may become very high. It is also thought that, when insulin does not work properly (insulin resistance), this fat is much more likely to be laid down in the liver.

'Fatty liver' is more common in children and young people with poorly controlled diabetes and sometimes the liver may become greatly enlarged. The only treatment is to improve control of the diabetes, following which the liver will steadily shrink back to its normal size.

Inheritance

My father had diabetes. Am I likely to get it too?

Diabetes is a common disorder in this country and is diagnosed
in about 3 in 100 people – in fact it probably affects about 5 in 100
people, because it hasn't been diagnosed yet. So in any large
family more than one person may be affected, simply by chance
alone. However, certain families do seem to carry a very strong
tendency for diabetes. The best example of this is a whole tribe of
Native Indians (the Pima): over half of its members develop
diabetes by the time they reach middle age.

Genes are the parts of a human cell that decide which characteristics you inherit from your parents. The particular genes that
you get from each parent are a matter of chance – in other words,
whether you grow up with your father's big feet or your mother's
blue eyes. Similarly it is a matter of chance whether you pass on
the genes carrying the tendency for diabetes to one of your children. It is *only* the tendency to diabetes that you may pass on –
the full-blown condition will *not* develop unless something else
causes the insulin cells in the pancreas to fail.

If diabetes is known to be in my family, should I or my children take any preventive action?

The inheritance of diabetes is a complicated subject – indeed
different sorts of diabetes appear to be inherited in different
ways. For instance, a tendency for one sort of diabetes (Type 1)
can be inherited, but only a small proportion of the people who
inherit this tendency will go on to develop diabetes. It is now
possible to tell if these people at risk have inherited the family of
relevant genes, and to a certain extent their chances of
developing diabetes can be predicted. In practice these tests are
only carried out when people are taking part in a research
project.

The more common Type 2 diabetes, often treated by diet or by
diet and tablets, is only rarely associated with known single gene
abnormality but it is thought to be strongly inherited in many

cases. Although there is a great deal more to learn about it, there may be several different subtypes which cannot be distinguished from one another – all inherited in different ways. We know that many of these people are overweight and that obesity not only makes diabetes worse but it may even lead to its appearance in susceptible people.

There is now evidence that family members who are at risk may put off developing diabetes by taking regular exercise and dieting to lose weight. They should have a blood glucose test as soon as they develop any relevant symptoms, so that the diabetes can be detected and treated early.

I am 16 and have had diabetes for 5 years. Why has my identical twin brother not got diabetes?

A large study has been carried out in which examples of identical twins with diabetes have been collected for over 20 years. These results show a difference between Type 1 and Type 2 diabetes. If you have an identical twin with Type 1 diabetes, you have only a 50% chance of developing diabetes yourself. On the other hand, if you had Type 2 diabetes (extremely unusual at the age of 11) your twin would be almost 100% certain to get the same sort of diabetes. In your case if your twin brother has not developed diabetes within the last 5 years, he has a very low risk of developing the condition.

2
Treatment without insulin

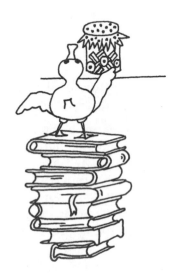

In this chapter and the next we describe different ways of treating diabetes. In younger people there is usually no choice and they need to start insulin injections fairly soon, but in older people found to have diabetes, the eventual form of treatment that they will need may not be obvious at the outset. Provided that they are not feeling terribly ill, they are usually given advice to change the type and quantity of food that they eat. This alone may have a dramatic effect on their condition, especially in overweight people who manage to get their weight down. If changing the diet fails to control diabetes, tablets are usually tried next by adding them to the diet. These may be very effective but tablets do not always work and in such cases insulin is the only alternative. Treatment with insulin is discussed in Chapter 3.

Knowing about the right type of food and the amount that you can eat is important. Most of the questions we have included help explain the general principles but people's diets are very individual, so do ask for help and further explanations from your own diabetes advisers and dietitians. It is particularly important to have an opportunity to review what you are doing about diet on a regular basis. If you are looking for new ideas for meals, there are now many helpful recipe books written especially for people with diabetes, most of which are available from Diabetes UK. A list of current titles can be found in Appendix 2.

Most people with diabetes, and especially parents who have a child with diabetes, long for a miracle cure. This explains why we have been sent so many questions about unorthodox methods of treatment. We have tried to answer these questions in a sensitive manner but there is no escaping the fact that, for a child, insulin is the only miracle cure and that is how it was regarded when it was discovered in 1921.

Diet

There must be many people like me who have diabetes but who are not on insulin. Why have I been told to control my weight?

People who develop diabetes later in life are often overweight. For the first few years after diagnosis, they do not usually need treatment with insulin injections – instead their treatment is by diet alone or by diet and tablets.

If you are overweight, the insulin produced by your pancreas is less effective because of the excess fat in your body. This is known as 'insulin resistance', and you overcome it by losing some of the fat. Achieving and maintaining a sensible weight therefore helps you improve control of your diabetes. An additional benefit is that it also reduces all the other health risks associated with being overweight, such as high blood pressure and heart disease.

I'm sure I don't eat too much. Why do I keep putting on weight?

Your body needs energy from food and drink to fuel your body processes, such as breathing, which go on even when you are sleeping. All forms of physical activity (such as walking, shopping, typing and so on) require additional energy. This energy is measured in calories or joules (see below).

Ideally your calorie intake from the food you eat should balance the amount of energy used by your body. When this happens you will neither gain nor lose weight. If the amount of food and drink you consume provides more energy (calories) than you use in your daily activities, then the extra food will be converted into body fat and you will put on weight. If you are overweight, you need to reduce your daily intake of calories so that you are taking in less energy than your body needs. Your body will make up the difference by using up the fat stored in your body and you will then lose weight.

In the UK we usually refer to calories, but some countries refer to joules: 1 calorie is equal to 4.2 joules. Strictly speaking, we should really be talking about kilocalories (often abbreviated to kcal) and kilojoules (abbreviated to kjoules or kJ), and these are the units that you will probably see on the nutritional information labels on food packaging. Most people simply use the shorthand term 'calorie' when they mean kilocalories, and this is what we have used in this book.

I have diabetes controlled by diet alone. Do I have to keep to strict mealtimes?

People on medication for diabetes (tablets or insulin) are usually advised to keep fairly closely to regular mealtimes to avoid getting a low blood sugar level (hypo). As long as you are on diet alone, your risk of a hypo is very low, so you do not need to keep to strict mealtimes. However, it is worth remembering that everyone finds their diabetes easier to control if they have three or more small meals a day rather than one or two large ones.

My husband's diabetes is controlled by diet alone. Since being diagnosed 2 years ago, he has kept strictly to his food plan. In the past year he has not had a positive urine test and his blood glucose measurements at the clinic have been normal. Does this mean he no longer has diabetes?

Once you have developed diabetes, you always have diabetes. This applies to almost everyone and exceptions to this are extremely rare. Your husband has obviously done very well by keeping to his food plan, and this is the reason his diabetes is so well controlled. If he went back to his old eating habits and started putting on weight, it is very likely that all his old symptoms would return and his blood glucose would be high again.

Do people on diet alone need to eat snacks in between meals?

No, not usually. The reason that people taking insulin injections are sometimes advised to eat a snack between their main meals is to balance the effect of the insulin they take. People on diet alone or diet and tablets do not usually have this problem and so do not usually need to have snacks. Of course snacks are not very helpful if you are trying to lose weight.

Remember that not eating snacks is not the same thing as missing meals. Some people on diet alone can go hypo if they go without food – there is a question about this in the section on *Hypos* in Chapter 3.

There seem to be many foods offered in the supermarkets now labelled 'diabetic foods'. Should I be eating these rather than the ordinary types?

No, and we would recommend that you do not even include them in your food plan. They are no lower in fats or calories than ordinary food and they are also expensive.

The main selling point for most of these so-called 'diabetic foods' is that they replace ordinary sugar with a substitute. This substitute may be another type of sugar called fructose, but is often a sugar alcohol called sorbitol. If taken in excess, this often leads to diarrhoea. Fructose and sorbitol both contain calories.

Today the recommended food plan for most people with diabetes allows you to include some sweetened foods, especially if you choose products with a higher fibre and lower fat content. If you are of normal weight or below, you will be able to eat modest amounts of ordinary extras or treats, such as biscuits, cakes or confectionery. These should form part of your food plan and should preferably be eaten at the end of a meal. There is therefore no need for you to buy diabetic foods just to give yourself a treat.

The only 'special' foods we recommend for people with diabetes are the ones labelled as 'diet' or 'low calorie', especially soft drinks that are sugar-free, reduced sugar preserves, diet yoghurts and sugar-free jellies. These are not marketed specifically for people with diabetes, but for everyone who wants to keep their weight under control or avoid eating too much sugar. They are usually sweetened with intense sweeteners such as saccharin or aspartame, which are virtually calorie-free. These artificial sweeteners can also be used to replace sugar in your tea or coffee, or you can get them in granular form to sprinkle on your breakfast cereal.

Where or how do I find out about the carbohydrate or calorie content of foods?

The publishers of the many slimming magazines on the market also produce booklets for slimmers listing the calorie contents of foods, and you may find that your local newsagent stocks one of these.

You could also look at the labels on the food you buy, as most foods are now labelled with their carbohydrate and calorie content (as well as with other nutritional information). Your dietitian can teach you how to use the information on these labels if you are not quite sure what something means. Some manufacturers label their foods more clearly than others.

I have just started tablets for my diabetes. Does this mean I can relax my diet?

Unfortunately not. You will have been prescribed tablets because treatment with diet alone was not enough to bring your blood glucose level down. If you start taking tablets and then relax your diet, your blood glucose levels may climb even higher. Remember, it's treatment with diet, exercise and tablets, not just with tablets.

If it has been a while since you have seen a dietitian, it would be a good idea to make an appointment to review your diet now that you are on tablets to see if there are any changes that you could make.

How does a person with diabetes get an appointment with a dietitian? Will there be one at my doctor's?

Everyone agrees that food plays a crucial part in the way people look after their diabetes. Soon after diagnosis and at other stages of diabetes, people need expert advice from a dietitian and this is recommended in the Diabetes UK booklet *What diabetes care to expect* (see Appendix 2). The availability of dietitians varies considerably across the country, but most diabetes centres have a dietitian as part of the team. Some general practitioners provide dietitian sessions in their own health centres, but in other places, you will have to wait for an appointment at the local hospital.

I have a number of queries about my diet. Can you tell me how I can get advice about it?

Good advice on diet is essential in the proper care of diabetes and it needs to be tailored to fit every individual person. Diabetes UK offers helpful literature and information but this is not really a substitute for personal advice from a properly trained dietitian.

You can arrange to see a State Registered Dietitian through your hospital or your GP. Most hospitals have a State Registered Dietitian attached to the diabetes clinic, and you could arrange to see them at your next clinic visit. Some general practitioners organize their own diabetes clinics, and may arrange for a dietitian to visit this clinic. Many nurses and health visitors who are specially trained in diabetes will also be able to provide good basic dietary advice.

I have many family celebrations in the summer and would like advice on the choice of alcoholic drinks. I have managed to lose weight and my control has improved so much that I have been taken off my tablets.

Taken in moderation, alcohol has been shown to be good for people with or without diabetes. You will need to remember that it can become a significant source of calories and can stimulate your appetite but, even on a weight-reducing diet, most people are allowed some alcohol for special occasions. As the control of your diabetes is so good, there will be no problem about enjoying a drink at your family celebrations.

You can choose from all types of wine, red or white, but should probably avoid very sweet wines and sherries on a regular basis because of their high sugar content. Spirits are sugar-free (but not calorie-free) and are best enjoyed with sugar-free ('diet' or 'slimline') mixers or soda water.

If you prefer a pint, you can choose beer, lager or cider. It is best to avoid the 'strong' brews, which are often labelled as being low in carbohydrate, as these are higher in alcohol and calories than the ordinary types. Low-alcohol and alcohol-free beers and lagers may contain a lot of sugar, so if you enjoy these you should look for the ones that are also labelled as being low in sugar.

Drinking alcohol affects your blood glucose level and you should be aware of this. You will find more information about this in the section on *Alcohol* in Chapter 5.

I have had diabetes for 22 years and have only recently come back under the care of my local hospital. When I talked about my diet to the dietitian she was keen to make some changes saying that there were quite a lot of new ideas and diet recommendations. What are these and is it worth me changing after all this time?

Advice on diet for people with diabetes has certainly changed since you were first diagnosed. Much more is now known about nutrition, and a diagnosis of diabetes no longer means eating differently from everyone else. In fact, the advice on a healthy diet for people with diabetes is exactly what has been recommended for the population as a whole – eating less fat, in particular saturated or animal fat, and sugar, and more fruit, vegetables and pulses. It's an eating plan that your whole family could follow if they want to eat healthily and well. Changing to a diet with more fruit and vegetables and less fat is certainly worthwhile and may reduce your risks of developing heart disease in later life.

We now know much more about carbohydrate, which is found in both sugary and starchy foods. In general, the carbohydrates found in sugary foods are more rapidly absorbed by the body, and make your blood glucose levels rise very quickly, which is not a good thing if you have diabetes. Starchy, high-fibre carbohydrate foods are absorbed more slowly and are more suitable because they make blood glucose levels rise more slowly. However, these days we rank carbohydrate foods in terms of their glycaemic index (GI). This is just a term to describe how slowly or quickly carbohydrate foods raise blood glucose levels. Foods that have a low glycaemic index like fruits, vegetables, pulses, pasta and rye bread should be combined with meals and snacks to help to control blood glucose levels, more easily. We give a list of foods in Table 2.1 with their GI numbers. Oat bran, for example, has a low glycaemic index. Low glycaemic index diets make insulin more responsive or 'sensitive' and this will help people with diabetes keep their blood sugar under control.

The dietary fibre found in these starchy carbohydrate foods is of two main types: 'fibrous' fibres, which are typically found in wholegrain cereals, wholemeal flour or bran; and 'viscous' fibres

Table 2.1 Glycaemic index of foods

FOOD	GI
Breakfast cereals	
All-Bran	42
Porridge	42
Special K	54
Muesli (variable)	56
Shredded Wheat	69
Weetabix	70
Cheerios	74
Puffed Wheat	74
Rice Krispies	82
Cornflakes	84
Bread	
Pumpernickel	41
Mixed grain	40–50
Pitta	57
Wholemeal	69
White	70
Baguette	95
Cereal grains	
Barley, whole or pearl	25
Rye	34
Bulgar	48
Barley, cracked	50
Buckwheat	54
Couscous	65
Millet	71
Rice	
Brown rice	55
Wild rice	57
Basmati rice	58
White rice, high-amylose	58
White rice, low-amylose	88
Instant rice (boiled 6 mins)	90

FOOD	GI
Pasta	
Fettucini	32
Vermicelli	35
Spaghetti, wholemeal	37
Spaghetti, white	41
Macaroni	45
Noodles, instant	47
Potatoes	
Sweet potato	54
New potato	62
Mashed potato	70
Instant potato	83
Baked potato	85
Pulses	
Beans:	
soya	18
kidney	27
butter	31
haricot	38
blackeye	42
baked	48
broad	79
Chick peas	33
Lentils	26–30
Peas:	
frozen (boiled)	48
dried (boiled)	22

found in pulses (peas, beans and lentils) and fruit and vegetables. Viscous fibres (especially those found in beans) appear to be of particular benefit because they slow down food absorption and hence the rate at which carbohydrate present in a meal will be absorbed into the bloodstream. All plant foods, especially those eaten raw or lightly cooked, are digested very slowly because the plant cell walls have to be broken down before their carbo-hydrate content is released. As well as this slow absorption (which means a slower rise in blood glucose levels), foods rich in fibre have a more prolonged effect on maintaining blood glucose levels. This reduces the risk of unexpected hypos if meals or snacks are delayed.

So it is worth updating your diet. Your dietitian will provide individual advice, but the main recommendations are summa-rized in the box (overleaf).

I am gradually losing my desire for sweet foods. When I do have them I follow my dietitian's advice and make sure that it is at a time when they are least likely to result in a high blood glucose. However, I really do not enjoy my selection of high-fibre breakfast cereals without some sweetener – I was a Sugar Puff fan before! Can I put a little sugar on?

Nowadays most experts accept that your food plan can include some sugar as part of a balanced diet. However, use one of the granulated sprinkle-type sweeteners, which are virtually calorie-free. Primarily aimed at slimmers, they are readily available in chemists and supermarkets. Brand names to look for include Canderel, Sweetex granulated, Sweet 'n' Low, and Hermesetas Sprinkle. These will not have any effect on your blood glucose.

Dietary advice for people with diabetes

- Eating too many *calories* in your diet will have a bad effect on control of your diabetes. Everyone with diabetes therefore requires a food and eating plan, based on their own individual needs, that does not contain a surplus food energy. (We have discussed balancing calories taken in and used up in more detail in the questions at the very beginning of this section.)

- To reduce your risk of developing coronary heart disease and arterial disease (and also to help you keep your weight under control) you should reduce the amount of saturated or animal *fat* in your diet. You can do this easily by substituting semi-skimmed or skimmed milk for whole milk; using less butter or margarine and replacing them with low fat spreads; reducing your intake of cream and cheese; grilling rather than frying foods; choosing fish, including two portions of oily fish per week, lean meat or poultry (skin removed). You should not eat too much protein and people with diabetes should probably avoid high protein/low carbohydrate diets.

- Although you should not add *sugar* to drinks, you can include foods containing sugar in your diet. You should base meals on *starchy carbohydrates*, like bread, pasta, rice, cereals and potatoes. Eat plenty of foods such as fruit, vegetables, pulses and beans. Breakfast cereals such as Weetabix, Shredded Wheat, Bran Flakes, All-Bran or porridge are all a good source of fibre.

- If you need to lose weight, you should not follow a diet low in *carbohydrate*: you should include some bread or potatoes, or pasta or rice, or breakfast cereal at each meal. A high carbohydrate/low fat diet is particularly suitable if you want to lose weight as it contains plenty of bulk and so you are less likely to feel hungry.

- Special '*diabetic foods*' are not worth including in your food plan because they are expensive and are usually high in calories. Low calorie '*diet foods*' and drinks that are sugar-free can be usefully included in your diet, especially if you need to lose weight. (We have talked about diabetic and diet foods in more detail in an earlier question.)

- You can drink a moderate amount of *alcohol* provided that you take its energy contribution (the number of calories it contains) into account. The recommended limit is 2 units per day for women and 3 units per day for men. One unit is the same as a glass of wine or sherry, a measure of spirits or ½ pint of beer, lager or cider. Beers and lagers specially brewed to be low in carbohydrate have a high alcohol and calorie content and are not recommended. (Again we have discussed this subject in more detail in an earlier question in this section.)

As a single parent I really find it hard to make ends meet. I know that very often I do not buy the foods that I should to help control my diabetes. Is there any way I can eat healthily but cheaply?

You are far from alone in wanting to eat well but cheaply nowadays. The sort of food plan advised for most people with diabetes should not cost more than the foods most people are eating before diagnosis, but there is no doubt that, when people are on very limited incomes, the amount they have to spend on food is often less than is required to buy a healthy diet. The following tips may help, and you could also ask your dietitian for some more ideas – it is a problem that will have often been met before.

For **breakfast**, have porridge, which is very cheap and an excellent breakfast cereal from the point of view of your diabetes control. When it's too hot for porridge, try home-made muesli, which you make by mixing some rolled oats (the type that you use to make porridge) with some fruit (perhaps a chopped apple) and some cold skimmed milk. You need enough milk to make the mixture about the same consistency as porridge, and you can also add some plain unsweetened low-fat yoghurt if you like. Leave it to stand overnight and it will be ready to eat in the morning.

A sandwich **lunch** can be very healthy, especially if you can use wholemeal bread. Tinned fish such as sardines, mackerel, or pilchards are excellent choices for sandwich fillings and can work out very inexpensive.

You do not really need large helpings of meat at your **main meals**, and you can often extend it with extra tinned, frozen or fresh vegetables. Diet yoghurts make excellent desserts and are good value for money. You can cut costs further by buying a large pot of plain natural yoghurt (usually cheaper than the fruit varieties) and adding chopped or puréed fresh or tinned fruit in natural juice with a little extra intense sweetener if needed. Another quick and healthy home-made dessert is a sugar-free jelly (available from most supermarkets) made up with milk or yoghurt.

The dietitian says that my high blood glucose levels during the morning may be caused by the pure fruit juice that I drink at breakfast. It is unsweetened juice, so how can this happen?

Pure unsweetened fruit juice will put up your blood glucose levels, whether it comes from a bottle or a carton or fresh fruit that you have squeezed yourself. All fruit contains natural sugar. If you eat it as the whole fruit then it takes time to be digested and the effect on blood glucose is quite slow. If you take away all the flesh (which contains the dietary fibre) and just drink the juice, the sugar will pass rapidly into your bloodstream.

You can have fruit juice but limit the amount you drink to a small glass. You can also dilute your fruit juice with mineral water or diet lemonade.

Overweight

I have just been told that I have diabetes. Is it true that if I lose weight I will probably not need insulin injections?

Possibly not, if you were overweight at the time of diagnosis, but as with many questions we have to qualify this by saying that it all depends on a number of factors.

Most of the people in the UK who have diabetes do not need insulin, especially those who are over 40 years old at the time of diagnosis and who are overweight. People who are of normal weight at the time of diagnosis are more likely to need treatment with insulin or with diet and tablets rather than just with diet alone. If you are overweight, it is impossible to predict how much weight you will need to lose in order to control your diabetes. In some people the loss of 3 kg (half a stone) is enough to restore the blood glucose to normal, while in other people the blood glucose remains high even after they lose many kilograms in weight. These people may then need tablets or insulin but, provided that they do not become too thin, they will still be better off for shedding the excess weight. Diabetes is, however, a progressive condition so, even if you can control it by diet alone initially, over time you will probably need tablet treatment and eventually insulin.

I am trying to lose weight. How much should I lose a week?

It depends on how much you weigh, how active you are, and what you were eating before you decided to tackle your weight problem. As a general rule people should be quite happy with a weight loss of anything between ½–1 kg (1–2 lbs) a week. This doesn't sound very much, especially when you can read about diets that claim to offer you a rapid weight loss of several kilograms a week. Losing weight slowly and steadily is healthier than losing weight very fast, which makes you lose muscle as well as fat. It is a common observation that people who lose weight too quickly tend to regain their previous weight and more within a few years.

Most people can lose weight by modifying the quantities and types of food they eat, particularly by cutting down the amounts of fat, sugar and alcohol. By 'saving' about 500 calories a day, they will lose about 1 lb (½ kg) a week. Increased exercise will also help to reduce weight. Even a small amount of weight loss will help to control your diabetes.

I have been dieting on and off since I had my last child 15 years ago. The diabetes that I developed in that pregnancy has now returned despite the fact that I don't take sugar in my drinks. What more can I do?

The answer probably lies in your dieting 'on and off'. If you are still overweight, you should try to reduce your energy (calorie) intake until you lose the excess weight. Once you have lost the weight, you will then need to follow a sensible eating plan that balances the amount of energy you take in with the amount you use up in your daily activities, and you will then be able to keep your weight steady.

To lose weight, try to concentrate on reducing the amount of fat that you eat, and cut down on foods that contain both fat and sugar, especially biscuits and confectionery. If this does not work, seek help from a dietitian who will take a dietary history and work out where else you can save calories. Finally, increasing the amount of regular exercise that you take can help.

Why are both my dietitian and diabetes specialist nurse so against my family buying me diabetic foods? I find my diet very hard to keep to and never lose weight anyway. So why can't I have diabetic foods as a treat?

In all probability the reason why you are not losing weight is that you are eating these 'diabetic foods' on top of your diet. Unfortunately foods labelled as 'diabetic' are often just as high in calories as standard versions. 'Diabetic' chocolate and biscuits contain just as many calories and just as much fat as the ordinary varieties so there is no real benefit.

I am very overweight and trying hard to lose about 20 kg (3 stone). I love ice cream and most of the cheaper varieties in the supermarket contain non-milk fat. Will this be suitable for me?

It would be acceptable to have a small bowl (1–2 scoops) of ice cream now and again, as part of your diet plan. Non-milk fat means that the manufacturers have used cheaper vegetable fats, which have just as many calories as milk fat. Most ice cream contains about 7–10% fat and around 80–100 calories per scoop – more in Cornish ice cream. You can buy reduced calorie ice cream but it is more expensive and the saving in calories does not really justify it for occasional use. Remember, ice cream is not an everyday food, anyway.

I have heard that there is a new appetite suppressant on the market but is it suitable for people with diabetes?

There is a new appetite suppressant which has been approved by a government body for use in diabetes. It goes by the name of sibutramine (Reductil) and may be given to people with diabetes, who are above a certain weight. Sibutramine is not suitable for everyone and should not be used in people with heart disease. You can continue to use the drug only if it leads to weight reduction of at least 2 kg (4 lbs) per month, and should not be considered as a long-term treatment.

I have the greatest difficulty losing weight and a friend has suggested that I should try joining 'Weight Watchers'. Will they accept people with diabetes?

'Weight Watchers' and similar slimming clubs can be very helpful to people who are having trouble losing weight, and that includes people with diabetes. They may ask for a letter from your doctor confirming that they have no objection. We frequently encourage people to join a slimming club, as they are often very successful in helping with weight loss where other efforts have failed and support you after you have reached your target weight and need to maintain your weight loss. Some people respond better to group therapy.

Exercise

I've heard that exercise is good for people with diabetes – is this true? If so, I'm not the 'sporty type' and have never found going to the gym has any appeal to me. What should I do?

Exercise is good for people with diabetes (and for everyone else as well), and indeed it is one of the few things that have been shown to actually reduce the risk of developing diabetes. Exercise does not have to involve sports, and you can usually find something suitable to suit your lifestyle. The staff at your local fitness centre are specially trained to help you with this, and these centres are a good place to start. They will work out an exercise programme with you and show you how to improve your fitness. Here are some ideas that you can adopt right away:

- Walk wherever you can and avoid using the car.
- Climb stairs rather than take the lift.
- Walk to and from work.
- Take your dog for more/longer walks.
- Consider buying a bicycle.
- Make a point of taking at least three half-hour walks a week at a fast pace.

If I keep to a good diet, why do I need to exercise as well?

Regular exercise stimulates a series of events in the body that results in changes in body composition and increased 'fitness'. Regular exercise increases the amount of lean tissue and reduces the amount of fat. Lean tissues consist of muscle, fibres and bone and all are enhanced by exercise. This increase in lean tissues increases your metabolic rate and the amount of exercise that you can do without getting tired/exhausted (fitness). This not only makes you feel better but it also reduces blood pressure and the 'bad' (low density) cholesterol and increases the 'good' (high density) cholesterol (see the next question about cholesterol). Increasing fitness also increases the body's sensitivity to insulin and lowers blood glucose levels. It may also increase the tendency to develop hypoglycaemia and you might have to reduce your insulin dose as your fitness improves.

I have been to have a cholesterol check-up, but I noted that the doctor also wanted to check for HDL and LDL. What's the difference between all these measurements and what are they?

Cholesterol is lipid (fat) and an important normal component of many body tissues. Its concentration in the blood, where it circulates attached to a protein (hence it is a 'lipoprotein'), has been shown to be a valuable indicator of the risk of developing vascular disease. High levels of cholesterol are associated with an increased risk of heart attacks. There are two major components of cholesterol known as low density lipoprotein (LDL) and high density lipoprotein (HDL). LDL is otherwise known as the 'bad' cholesterol as it is the most important risk factor for heart disease. HDL on the other hand is the 'good' cholesterol, since high levels of HDL are associated with a low risk of heart disease. Thus a 'high cholesterol value' is ambiguous unless you know whether it is high because of increased LDL or HDL cholesterol. This is important as HDL values are often high in people with Type 1 diabetes (insulin raises the HDL level) and as such do not indicate an increased risk of heart disease. Thus before contemplating any treatment for a 'high cholesterol', your doctor needs to know that it is the 'bad' cholesterol (LDL) that is to blame. It's a complicated story and we hope that this explanation helps? For those who seek more information, have a look at:

http://www.lipidsonline.org/slides/slide01.cfm?tk=9

I have Type 2 diabetes and take the highest doses of metformin and gliclazide but am not well controlled. My doctor tells me that I could avoid insulin if I made a determined effort to improve my fitness and lose some weight. Is this true?

Yes, your doctor is right. It has been clearly shown that exercise can improve metabolic control in people with poorly-controlled Type 2 diabetes. If you are to succeed, you will need to adopt a fitness programme and continue this on a regular basis. If you wish to lose weight as well, you will need to combine this exercise programme with a calorie-reduced diet, as exercise by itself is not a good way of losing weight. If you want to pursue this line, we suggest you go along to your local fitness centre and sign up with a 'Personal Trainer' who will give you a suitable programme, encourage you and monitor your progress.

Tablets

I understand that there are different sorts of 'diabetic' tablets. Can you tell me what they are and what the difference is between them?

There are five different types of tablets that may be prescribed for people with diabetes. They work in different ways.

- *Sulphonylureas* (including gliclazide, chlorpropamide, glibenclamide, glipizide, glimepiride, gliquidone and tolbutamide): they act by increasing the amount of natural insulin produced by your pancreas.
- *Biguanide* (metformin [Glucophage]): this works by reducing the release of glucose from your liver and increasing the uptake of glucose into muscle.
- *Alpha glucosidase inhibitor* (acarbose [Glucobay]): this slows the digestion of carbohydrates in your intestine and suppresses the rise in blood glucose after meals.
- *Thiazolidenediones* (rosiglitazone [Avandia] and pioglitazone [Actos]): they target 'insulin resistance' and are used in people who have been unable to control their blood glucose levels with metformin or a sulphonylurea. Rosiglitazone is also available in combination with metformin (Avandamet).
- *Prandial glucose regulators* (repaglinide and nateglinide): these stimulate the release of insulin from your pancreas and are given with meals (prandial means a meal). They can be used on their own or combined with metformin.

I am taking gliclazide but am getting dizziness. Could the tablets be causing this?

Gliclazide could be causing your blood glucose level to be too low so your dizziness could be a mild hypo, particularly if you get this feeling when exercising or before meals. You can easily confirm this by checking your blood glucose at a time when you feel dizzy. If your blood glucose level is above 4 mmol/litre then something apart from the gliclazide must be causing the dizziness. There are of course other causes of dizziness, which have nothing to do with diabetes, and your doctor will check for these.

I find I am dropping off to sleep all the time and never feel refreshed. I take 160 mg of gliclazide twice a day as well as 500 mg metformin. Could I be taking too much?

This is quite a large dose of gliclazide and your sleepiness could be due to a hypo. You should check that your blood glucose is not too low (below 4 mmol/litre). On the other hand, people with a high blood glucose often feel drowsy and lacking in energy. So your complaint could be due to either a low or a high blood glucose level, and you can find out by doing a blood glucose test. Take the results to your doctor who will adjust your dose accordingly if necessary.

My doctor is taking me off Diabinese (chlorpropamide). Will I get withdrawal symptoms?

Some medicines, especially certain sleeping tablets and painkillers, become necessary to the body if taken regularly for long periods of time. When these drugs are stopped, the body reacts violently, causing withdrawal symptoms. Tablets for diabetes do not have these effects and can be stopped quite safely – provided, of course, that you no longer need them to keep your blood glucose under control. If your blood glucose begins to rise, the symptoms of thirst, itching, and so on, will return, but these cannot be described as withdrawal symptoms. They are due to the diabetes returning.

Since taking Glucophage (metformin), I have had feelings of nausea and constant diarrhoea and have lost quite a lot of weight. Is this due to the Glucophage?

Nausea and diarrhoea are possible side effects of Glucophage. The loss of weight could be due either to poor food intake because Glucophage has reduced your appetite, or to your diabetes being out of control. Either way you should stop

Glucophage or at least reduce the dose and see if the nausea and diarrhoea disappear. If your diabetes is then poorly controlled with high blood glucose levels (more than 10 mmol/litre), you may need a different sort of tablet or perhaps insulin injections in addition to diet, and you should consult your doctor.

My elderly mother has been taking gliclazide to control her diabetes for 5 years. Recently her sugars have been high and her doctor has asked her to take metformin as well with good results. Are there concerns about the long-term safety of metformin?

Metformin is a very good drug and we are not surprised that your mother's diabetic control has been better since she started taking it in addition to gliclazide. The down side is that metformin frequently causes side effects, mainly affecting the stomach or digestion (diarrhoea, constipation, nausea, loss of appetite). These side effects may develop after metformin has been taken for several years.

What is the cause of a continuous metallic burning taste in the mouth? I am 62 years of age with diabetes, controlled on tablets for the last 4 years.

You are probably taking metformin (Glucophage) tablets as these sometimes do cause a curious taste in the mouth. If the taste is troublesome (and it sounds unpleasant) you should stop taking these tablets. Other tablets for diabetes do not cause this side effect. You should consult your doctor for advice.

I have diabetes controlled on tablets. My dose was halved, and my urine was still negative to glucose. Would it be all right to stop taking my tablets altogether to see what happens? Obviously I would restart the tablets if my urine showed glucose.

Your idea is probably a good one, but you should discuss this with your doctor. You should also check your blood glucose level as urine tests can sometimes be misleading. Provided that your blood glucose remains controlled (less than 8 mmol/litre) you would be better off finding out if you can control your blood glucose without any tablets. If you no longer need tablets, diet becomes even more important for controlling your diabetes and you must avoid putting on weight. Some people think that if they come off tablets, they no longer have diabetes, but this is not so. There is always the chance that they will need tablets or even insulin at some stage in the future.

I have just started taking Glucobay tablets for my diabetes. Could you explain how Glucobay works?

Glucobay, the trade name for acarbose, acts by slowing the digestion of starch and related foodstuffs. Acarbose (Glucobay) slows the breakdown and absorption of many dietary carbohydrates, reducing the high peak of blood glucose which can occur after eating a meal containing carbohydrate. It was launched in the UK in 1993, having been used very extensively in other European countries. It is an addition to diet treatment and has been shown to be effective in many people with diabetes who do not require insulin treatment.

I take Glucobay tablets but always feel very full and bloated afterwards. Would it be better not to take them?

Acarbose (Glucobay) may lead to side effects when you first start taking it. These side effects are related to its action in the body (see the previous question). Because Glucobay slows down the breakdown of carbohydrates, complex sugars may then reach the lower part of the gut where they can cause a bloating sensation giving rise to wind (flatulence) and occasional transient diarrhoea. There are two ways of reducing this problem.

Start with a very small dose of one 50 mg tablet of Glucobay a day, taken with the first mouthful of your largest meal. Increase the dose slowly, in consultation with your doctor, until the optimum dose is reached. This may be up to 100 mg three times a day.

Try and exclude sucrose from your diet. Sucrose is the ordinary sugar that we add knowingly to sweeten food. It is also added to many foodstuffs by the manufacturers.

I have heard that there is an anti-obesity pill that works by stopping fat absorption. Would it be suitable for me? I have diabetes and am very overweight.

The tablet you are probably referring to is called Xenical, the brand name for orlistat. It blocks the digestion of fat and is the first anti-obesity pill not to rely on suppressing appetite. Orlistat manipulates the chemical digestion processes, blocking the action of lipases (enzymes that break up fat in the intestine), so that about 30% of fat in any meal goes undigested. However, there can be unpleasant side effects. The dietary fat that is not absorbed can be rapidly excreted, which can lead to stomach cramps, diarrhoea and leakage of faeces. Many nutritionists credit the drug's success to these side effects as they encourage adherence to a low fat diet. There is no reason why a person with diabetes cannot take orlistat, but you should discuss this with your health professional.

I gather that there is a new 'type' of tablet for the treatment of diabetes called 'rosiglitazone'. What's different about it?

Rosiglitazone (trade name Avandia, or Avandamet in combination with metformin, from GlaxoSmithKline) is an entirely new form of medication designed for people with Type 2 diabetes. It acts by reducing the body's resistance to insulin. It has been tested extensively in the UK and elsewhere in clinical trials in people with Type 2 diabetes, and is recommended as an additional therapy in combination with either metformin or a sulphonylurea (e.g. gliclazide or glibenclamide) when metabolic control is not adequate. The newly formed NHS National Institute of Clinical Excellence (NICE) has reviewed all the information available on the drug and has recently given it their 'seal of approval'. Because it is a new drug, certain precautions with its use are advised.

I am a 65-year-old and remain a bit overweight despite my best efforts to reduce my weight through strict dieting and increasing the amount of exercise I take. I know my metabolic control is not good and I am on what my doctor says is a maximum dose of metformin. Today she suggested I add a new tablet called 'pioglitazone' to my treatment. She says that it is a new type of tablet and, because of this, I will need to have a blood test to check on my liver. This all sounds a bit formidable – should I go ahead and try these new tablets?

It sounds as if your doctor is giving you sound advice. Pioglitazone is a relatively new drug and trials have shown it to be effective and safe in improving metabolic control in people such as yourself. However, because it should not be used in people with liver problems, an initial liver blood test is advised, with follow-up blood tests each year.

I am about to go onto a glitazone and would like to know how it works.

You probably have Type 2 diabetes (see Chapter 1) that is not well controlled on your present tablets. Rosiglitazone was introduced in 1999 and relies on the fact that Type 2 diabetes is caused by failure to produce insulin *and* resistance to the insulin that is available. Glitazones work by making you more sensitive to insulin so that whatever you can produce goes further. Troglitazone was the first of this group of drugs to reach the market but it caused serious liver problems in a few people and had to be withdrawn. Extensive tests have been done on the new glitazones (rosiglitazone and pioglitazone) and they appear to be completely safe. However, most doctors like to arrange liver function tests when they first start people on these drugs.

Glitazones may be used as initial treatment in people who cannot tolerate metformin, or added to metformin, particularly if they are overweight. Rosiglitazone may also be used with metformin and a sulphonylurea.

Unlike other drugs used for diabetes, glitazones work slowly and may take up to 3 months to have their full effect.

I've just been put on pioglitazone and my blood glucose readings are no better – should I stop taking it?

Pioglitazone, like rosiglitazone, can be an effective way of controlling Type 2 diabetes. However, it does not usually have a rapid effect and you should wait 3 months before concluding that it is not helping your blood sugars.

I'm on rosiglitazone and gliclazide and my doctor wants to put me on metformin as well. Is this OK?

Yes, rosiglitazone has recently been licensed for use in triple combination treatment with metformin and a sulphonylurea. Presumably your blood sugars are running high on your present tablets and your doctor is adding in metformin as a last ditch attempt to avoid the need for insulin. The chances of success are only around 70% but it is worth giving it a try if there is a very good reason for avoiding insulin (e.g. you may hold an HGV licence – see the section on *Driving* in Chapter 5).

My doctor has recently started me on Novonorm, which I understand is a new type of tablet for diabetes. How does it differ from metformin, which I also take?

Novonorm is the trade name for repaglinide, which is a prandial glucose regulator. This means that it controls the high glucose levels that can occur when food is consumed. It is a blood glucose-lowering tablet that stimulates the quick release of insulin from your pancreas at mealtimes, and should be taken just before a meal. If a meal is missed, the repaglinide is not taken (unlike metformin). Nateglinide (trade name Starlix) is another prandial glucose regulator. These tablets are usually used in combination with metformin.

I take a lot of tablets and have been told that I will probably have to change to insulin soon. What is the maximum dose of tablets I could take before insulin is required?

We have listed the minimum and maximum doses of tablets that you can take each day in Table 2.2.

Many people continue to use the maximum dose of tablets for years with rather poor control of their diabetes (blood glucose consistently greater than 10 mmol/litre). Although these people often feel fairly well in themselves, they are usually much better off when they change to insulin. After the change to insulin people notice that they have more energy and can usually manage on a less strict diet. In addition, running high blood sugar levels for years carries an increased risk of heart disease and other diabetic complications, such as eye problems (see the section on *Eyes* in Chapter 9.

What should I do if I am ill while on tablets? Should I take more or perhaps fewer tablets?

During the illness, you may not feel like eating, but you must not stop your tablets as any illness usually causes the blood glucose to rise. If your blood glucose readings become very high, you should contact your GP.

My doctor has advised me to change from tablets to insulin. Would I be right in thinking that I could avoid doing this if I cut down my intake of carbohydrate?

No, probably not. If you are overweight, you *might* be able to avoid insulin by dieting strictly and losing weight but only if you are eating more than you need at the moment. If your present food intake is the amount you need, then reducing this will only make you lose weight and in due course become weak – and you may already be suffering from thirst, weight loss and fatigue. So if you are eating too much, eat less and try to improve your control that way. If you are already dieting properly, do not try to

Table 2.2 Diabetes tablets

Name	Trade name	Dose range (mg)
Sulphonylureas *(taken once or twice daily)*		
chlorpropamide	no longer recommended	
glibenclamide	Daonil, Semi-Daonil, Euglucon, Diabetamide, Gliken	2.5–15
gliclazide	Diamicron, Diaglyk	40–320
glipizide	Glibenese, Minodiab	2.5–40
glimepiride	Amaryl	1–6
gliquidone	Glurenorm	15–180
tolbutamide	Rastinon	500–2000
Biguanide *(taken 2–3 times daily)*		
metformin	Glucophage	500–3000
Alpha glucosidase inhibitor *(taken 3 times daily)*		
acarbose	Glucobay	50–600
Thiazolidenedione *(taken 1–2 times daily)*		
rosiglitazone	Avandia	4–8
rosiglitazone/metformin	Avandamet combination	2/1000–8/2000
pioglitazone	Actos	15–30
Prandial glucose regulators *(taken up to 4 times daily)*		
repaglinide	NovoNorm	0.5–16
nateglinide	Starlix	60–360

starve yourself. Accept insulin and you will probably be grateful, especially if it makes you feel better and more energetic.

My diabetes has been treated with tablets for 2 years and now my doctor has said I need insulin injections. Is my diabetes getting worse?

If your blood glucose can no longer be controlled with tablets, then your pancreas is becoming even less efficient in producing insulin, and in that sense your diabetes is worse. However, it does not mean that you are going to suffer any new problems from the condition, nor does it necessarily mean that you have done anything wrong. Diabetes is a progressive condition and many people will eventually move on to insulin. Once you have got over the initial fear of injecting yourself (and most people manage this very quickly), then going on to insulin should not alter your life – in fact it will probably make you feel much better.

My mother is quite elderly and may have to take insulin. Are there new ways of giving insulin that will make it simpler for her?

We agree that new insulin devices (Innolet) have made it easier for old people to administer insulin. However, it is often difficult to predict whether an older person will be better off on insulin rather than tablets. The factors that her doctor will take into consideration are as follows:

- How unwell or thirsty does she feel while on tablets?
- What side effects are the tablets causing?
- How high are her blood sugars?
- How active and dexterous is she?
- How keen is she to start insulin?

Of all these questions, the last one is the most important and we must not pressurize older people to start a form of treatment, which they may dread. One way round this is to try insulin for a specified period of say 2 months and allow her to decide after that time whether or not she wishes to continue with insulin or revert to her previous treatment with tablets.

Non-medical treatments

Recently I saw a physical training expert demonstrating a technique of achieving complete relaxation. She concluded by saying 'Of course, this is not suitable for everyone, for example people with diabetes'. Is this true and, if so, why?

This sounds like an example of ignorant discrimination. There is no reason why people with diabetes should not practise complete relaxation if they want to. If the session went on for a long time, you might have to miss a snack or even a meal but as you are burning up so little energy in a relaxed state, it should not matter.

My back has troubled me for many years and a friend has suggested that as a last resort I should try acupuncture. Would there be any objection to this, given that I have diabetes? Might it even help my diabetes?

Acupuncture has been a standard form of medical treatment in China for 5000 years. In the last 20 years it has become more widely used in this country. In China acupuncture has always been thought of as a way of preventing disease and is considered less effective in treating illness. In the UK acupuncture tends to be used by people who have been ill (and usually in pain) for a long time. It is most often tried in such conditions as a painful back, where orthodox medicine has failed to help. Even practitioners of the art do not claim that acupuncture can cure diabetes, but it will not do it any harm either, provided that you do not alter your usual diabetes treatment while you are having your course of acupuncture. If you have neuropathy (see Chapter 9) and have little sensation, it may be sensible to avoid acupuncture in the affected areas.

Do you think that complementary or alternative medicine can help people with diabetes?

Alternative medicine suggests a form of treatment that is taken in the place of conventional medical treatment. As such this could potentially be very dangerous, particularly if your diabetes is treated with insulin.

However, there may be a place for complementary therapies that can be tried alongside conventional medicine. Although there is no scientific evidence to show that complementary therapies such as yoga, reflexology, hypnosis or aromatherapy can benefit someone with diabetes, some people who have tried them report that they feel more relaxed. As stress can have a detrimental effect on blood glucose control, it may mean that their diabetes improves as a result.

We must emphasize that these therapies should always be used in addition to, not instead of, your usual diabetes treatment. You should not alter your recommended diet or stop taking your tablets or your insulin, nor would a reputable complementary practitioner suggest that you do any of these things.

I have heard that there are herbal remedies for diabetes. What would these be?

There are many plants that have been said to reduce the high level of blood glucose in people with diabetes. One of these is a berry from West Africa and another a tropical plant called karela or bitter gourd. The problem is that to get any significant effect you need to consume more karela than is realistic. Consequently, it has only a minimal effect on lowering blood glucose and, as the bitter gourd lives up to its name and tastes disgusting, you will find conventional tablets more convenient, more reliable and safer. Herbal remedies have no effect on diabetes that requires insulin treatment.

I recently read an article on ginseng that said it was beneficial to people with diabetes. Have you any information on this?

Ginseng comes from Korea and the powdered root is said to have amazing properties. There is no scientific evidence to suggest that it is of any help to people with diabetes.

My little girl has just contracted diabetes at the age of 3. I would do anything to cure her. Would hypnosis be worth a try?

Most parents are desperate for a cure when their child develops diabetes. In one sense, insulin injections are a cure in that they replace the missing hormone, but this is not much consolation to a distressed parent. Although a sense of desperation is natural, it is best for your child's sake for you to try to accept that she will always have diabetes. In this way she is more likely to come to terms with the condition herself. It is normal to grieve but at some stage you must face facts as a family and make use of all the help that is available for you and your daughter. In that way she will be less upset about her diabetes than you are. Hypnosis will not help her insulin cells to regenerate.

An evangelistic healing crusade claims to heal among other diseases 'sugar diabetes', malignant growth and multiple sclerosis, etc. Are these claims correct?

There are, of course, a handful of (unproven) reports of miracle cures of various serious diseases like cancer, but these are few and far between. A mildly overweight person might be persuaded to lose weight by a faith healer and so it might appear that the diabetes was 'cured', but no person on insulin has ever benefited from a healing crusade except in the strictly spiritual sense.

3
Treatment with insulin

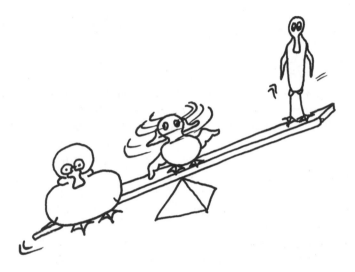

Insulin was discovered by Frederick Banting and Charles Best in the summer of 1921. The work was carried out in the Physiology Department of Toronto University while most of the staff were on their holidays. The first human to be given insulin was a 14-year-old boy named Leonard Thompson who was dying of diabetes in Toronto General Hospital. This was an historic event, representing the beginning of modern treatment for diabetes. It was then up to the chemists to transform the production of insulin into an industrial process on a vast scale.

When Dr Robin Lawrence heard the news, he was in Florence waiting to die from diabetes. Instead he lived on and, with H. G. Wells, went on to found the British Diabetic Association, now called Diabetes UK.

Insulin treatment replaces the insulin normally produced by the pancreas gland, which becomes severely deficient in most people whose diabetes develops before they are 30 years old. In people in whom diabetes develops later in life, the deficiency of insulin is much less marked and forms of treatment other than insulin injections usually work for some time, though usually not indefinitely. Treatment without insulin is covered in Chapter 2.

Insulin still has to be given by injection because at present it is inactivated if taken by mouth. Research is being carried out on inhaled and oral (by mouth) insulin, although neither treatment is available yet. About a quarter of all people with diabetes are treated with insulin. Virtually everyone who develops diabetes when they are young needs insulin from the time of diagnosis. People diagnosed in later life may manage quite satisfactorily for many years on other forms of treatment but eventually many of them will need insulin to supplement their diminishing supply of insulin from their pancreas.

Everyone dreads the thought of having to inject themselves but the modern needles and syringes or insulin pens are so good that in nearly all cases this fear disappears after the first few injections, and daily injections become no more of a hassle than brushing your teeth.

People on insulin still have to watch what they eat. There is a section on *Diet and insulin* in this chapter, but we suggest that you also read the section on *Diet* in Chapter 2, as the information there is relevant whatever your form of treatment. However, healthy eating is only part of the treatment. Being the right weight and getting enough exercise is also very important. There is a section on *Sports* in Chapter 5 we suggest you refer to.

The section on *Hypos* (low blood glucose) is one of the most important parts of this book. They usually affect people on insulin but can happen to those taking certain tablets. It is the fear of hypos that prevents some people from controlling their blood glucose tightly. Diabetes care teams are often criticized for not giving people who are newly diagnosed enough information on hypos. So if you have just started insulin treatment, read this section carefully.

Types of insulin

Since the discovery of insulin, countless people with diabetes have injected themselves with insulin extracted from the pancreas of cows and pigs. In the last 20 years or so human insulin has become widely available. However, human insulin is not extracted from human pancreas in the same way beef or pork insulin is. A great deal of research went into producing 'human' insulin by means of genetic engineering. This means that the genetic material of a bacterium or a yeast is reprogrammed to make insulin instead of the proteins it would normally produce. The insulin manufactured in this way is rigorously purified and contains no trace of the original bacterium.

The first insulin to be made was clear soluble insulin also called short-acting insulin. Injected under the skin, this insulin has a relatively rapid onset of action and lasts for 4–8 hours. Various modifications were made to this original insulin so that it would last longer after injection. When protamine or zinc is incorporated into the soluble insulin, a single injection could last from 12 to 36 hours. For many years a single daily injection was advised by doctors but people realized that this was not a good way of controlling the variations in blood glucose that occur during the day. Nowadays many people who need insulin have a mixture of short- and intermediate- or long-acting insulin twice a day, but an increasing number have insulin four or more times a day that they can inject with an insulin pen (see the section on *Insulin pens* later in this chapter). A new generation of insulins, also called insulin analogues, where the chemical make up of the insulin is changed, are also available today. By changing the molecular structure of the insulin, manufacturers can alter the way it works, allowing it to be absorbed differently.

I have been on ordinary pork insulin for 12 years and my doctor has just changed me over to human insulin. I feel upset because I was given no real explanation. Can you please help?

There has been a gradual switch to human insulin since it was introduced in 1982. Many doctors felt that human insulin was generally better because it led to less antibody formation than pork insulin. However, these antibodies probably do no harm and they may even be of some benefit by making the insulin injection last longer. There are also commercial pressures as insulin manufacturers would prefer to make only the human variety, which would in turn reduce production costs.

Most people are able to swap from animal to human insulin without any difficulty but it is usual to reduce the dose by about 10% to be on the safe side and to compensate for the reduction in antibodies. This may be a gradual process lasting up to 6 weeks. Obviously during this transition period you will need to be especially careful to do frequent blood checks and if necessary to adjust the dose of insulin.

If the new type of insulin causes any problems, you can always ask to go back on pork insulin.

Since changing to human insulin my hypos have changed. There is less warning and on several occasions I needed help from my wife to get me back to normal. Have other people had the same experience?

This is a fairly common complaint and is very worrying because people rely on their warning signs to help them cope with the problem of hypos. Before human insulin was introduced, exhaustive tests were performed to try and find ways in which it differed from animal insulin. In conclusion, these tests failed to show any significant differences apart from the lower levels of antibodies to insulin. It came as a surprise when a few people reported that their hypos were different on the new insulin and no real explanation has been found for this observation, but you may find it worthwhile to try the pork insulin again. (Please see the section on **Hypos** later in this chapter for more information.)

A self-help group exists for people who are treated with insulin, and their carers. The Insulin Dependent Diabetes Trust has highlighted a number of problems connected with insulin and the delivery of care. It has been an effective pressure group over the question of human insulin. See Appendix 3 for details.

I have had problems with human insulin and would like to go back to pork insulin. However, my chemist tells me that Velosulin is only available in the human form. Any suggestions?

It is true that pork Velosulin is no longer manufactured. However, the same company still makes Actrapid in both pork and human form. This is a highly purified soluble insulin comparable to Velosulin. You should be able to substitute porcine Actrapid for your original dose of porcine Velosulin. Alternatively, there are other companies like CP Pharmaceuticals who manufacture animal insulins exclusively.

There is no pork zinc insulin the same as Monotard, but Insulatard is often a good substitute, and this is available in both human or pork forms. For the record, Mixtard 30, a premixed solution of short and intermediate acting insulin, is also available in both forms. Cartridges for the insulin pen are available as human, bovine, or porcine insulin (see the list of insulins in Table 3.1).

My diabetes has been well controlled on beef insulin (soluble and isophane) for the past 22 years. Should I use human insulin instead?

Provided that you are doing well on your present insulin, there is no need to change. Although the major insulin companies have not made beef insulin for many years, a firm called CP Pharmaceuticals supplies beef and pork insulin under the brand names Hypurin Bovine and Hypurin Porcine. They produce short-acting insulin: Hypurin Bovine Neutral and Hypurin Porcine Neutral; intermediate-acting insulin: Hypurin Bovine Isophane and Hypurin Porcine Isophane; long-acting insulin: Hypurin Bovine

Table 3.1 Insulins available

Rapid-acting Insulin (analogue), which is clear, has an onset of action within 15 minutes, a peak action of 30–70 minutes, and lasts 2–5 hours

Name	Manufacturer	Source	Vial or cartridge
Humalog	Lilly	analogue	vial & cartridge
Humalog Pen	Lilly	analogue	preloaded pen
NovoRapid	Novo Nordisk	analogue	vial
NovoRapid Penfill*	Novo Nordisk	analogue	cartridge
NovoRapid FlexPen	Novo Nordisk	analogue	preloaded pen

Soluble Insulin, which is clear and lasts from 4–6 hours with a peak action at 2–3 hours

Name	Manufacturer	Source	Vial or cartridge
Human Actrapid	Novo Nordisk	human	vial
Actrapid FlexPen	Novo Nordisk	human	preloaded pen
Actrapid Penfill*	Novo Nordisk	human	cartridge
Human Velosulin	Novo Nordisk	human	vial
Pork Actrapid	Novo Nordisk	pork	vial
Humulin S	Lilly	human	vial & cartridge
Humaject S	Lilly	human	preloaded pen
Hypurin Porcine Neutral[†]	CP Pharmaceuticals	pork	vial & cartridge
Hypurin Bovine Neutral[†]	CP Pharmaceuticals	beef	vial & cartridge
Insuman Rapid	Aventis Pharma	human	vial & cartridge
Insuman Rapid Optiset	Aventis Pharma	human	preloaded pen

Intermediate- and Long-acting Insulin, which is cloudy and lasts 6–24 hours with a peak at 8–12 hours

Name	Manufacturer	Source	Vial or cartridge
Human Insulatard	Novo Nordisk	human	vial
Human Insulatard Penfill*	Novo Nordisk	human	cartridge
Human Insulatard FlexPen	Novo Nordisk	human	preloaded pen
Pork Insulatard	Novo Nordisk	pork	vial
Human Monotard	Novo Nordisk	human	vial
Human Ultratard	Novo Nordisk	human	vial
Levimir (insulin detemir)	Novo Nordisk	analogue	preloaded pen
Humulin I	Lilly	human	vial & cartridge
Humulin I Pen	Lilly	human	preloaded pen
Humulin Lente	Lilly	human	vial
Humulin ZN	Lilly	human	vial
Hypurin Porcine Isophane†	CP Pharmaceuticals	pork	vial & cartridge
Hypurin Bovine Isophane†	CP Pharmaceuticals	beef	vial & cartridge
Hypurin Bovine Lente†	CP Pharmaceuticals	beef	vial
Hypurin Bovine PZI†	CP Pharmaceuticals	beef	vial
Insuman Basal	Aventis Pharma	human	vial & cartridge
Insuman Basal Optiset	Aventis Pharma	human	preloaded pen
Lantus‡ (insulin glargine)§	Aventis Pharma	analogue	vial & cartridge
Lantus‡ Optiset	Aventis Pharma	analogue	preloaded pen

Table 3.1 Continued

Mixed Insulin containing both short- and longer-acting insulin. This is designed to have an early peak of action at 2 hours with a total action of more than 8 hours

Name	Manufacturer	Source	Vial or cartridge
Human Mixtard 30^{ll}	Novo Nordisk	human	vial
Pork Mixtard 30^{ll}	Novo Nordisk	pork	vial
Human Mixtard 10^{ll} Pen	Novo Nordisk	human	preloaded pen
Human Mixtard 20^{ll} Pen	Novo Nordisk	human	preloaded pen
Human Mixtard 30^{ll} Pen	Novo Nordisk	human	preloaded pen
Human Mixtard 40^{ll} Pen	Novo Nordisk	human	preloaded pen
Human Mixtard 50^{ll} Pen	Novo Nordisk	human	preloaded pen
Mixtard 10^{ll} Penfill*	Novo Nordisk	human	cartridge
Mixtard 20^{ll} Penfill*	Novo Nordisk	human	cartridge
Mixtard 30^{ll} Penfill*	Novo Nordisk	human	cartridge
Mixtard 40^{ll} Penfill*	Novo Nordisk	human	cartridge
Mixtard 50^{ll} Penfill*	Novo Nordisk	human	cartridge
Human Mixtard 50^{ll}	Novo Nordisk	human	vial
NovoMix 30 Penfill*¶	Novo Nordisk	analogue	cartridge
NovoMix 30 FlexPen¶	Novo Nordisk	analogue	preloaded pen
Humulin M2 20/80^{ll}	Lilly	human	cartridge
Humulin M3 30/70^{ll}	Lilly	human	vial & cartridge
Humulin M5	Lilly	human	vial
Humaject M3	Lilly	human	preloaded pen
Humalog Mix 25**	Lilly	analogue	cartridge & preloaded pen

56

Name	Manufacturer	Source	Vial or cartridge
Humalog Mix 50**	Lilly	analogue	preloaded pen
Insuman Comb 15||	Aventis Pharma	human	vial &cartridge
Insuman Comb 15 Optiset||	Aventis Pharma	human	preloaded pen
Insuman Comb 25||	Aventis Pharma	human	vial & cartridge
Insuman Comb 25 Optiset||	Aventis Pharma	human	preloaded pen
Insuman Comb 50||	Aventis Pharma	human	vial & cartridge
Insuman Comb 50 Optiset||	Aventis Pharma	human	preloaded pen
Hypurin Porcine† 30/70|| mix	CP Pharmaceuticals	pork	vial & cartridge

* All Novo Nordisk Penfills are available in 1.5 and 3.0 ml sizes
† All Hypurin packaging is marked with Braille
‡ Lantus and detemir are clear, not cloudy
§ Glargine is a basal analogue insulin (lasting 24 hours)
|| The numbers refer to the percentage of soluble (short-acting) to isophane (intermediate-acting) insulin, e.g. Mixtard 20 is 20% soluble to 80% isophane, Humulin M3 30/70 is 30% soluble to 70% isophane
¶ NovoMix 30 is 30% soluble insulin aspart and 70% insulin aspart protamine
*= Humalog mixes are a mixture of lispro solution and lispro protamine suspension (both analogue insulins)

Lente and Hypurin Bovine PZI; and also premixed insulin: Hypurin Porcine 30/70. All of these except Lente and PZI are available in cartridges as well as vials.

I have been taking beef insulin for many years and am worried about the possibility of this insulin being contaminated with BSE. Is this possible?

The manufacturers of beef insulin consider that the risk of any BSE (bovine spongiform encephalopathy) agent remaining after the intensive purification processes used to extract insulin is either negligible or non-existent. In addition, beef insulin used in the UK is derived from cattle originating in countries considered to have a negligible incidence of BSE, so that the risk of coming into contact with BSE through beef insulin is very small indeed.

I have seen a programme on television, which says that human insulin may be dangerous. My 14-year-old son has just developed diabetes and I see that the doctor has put him on human insulin. You can imagine how worried I am about it.

Yes, it is unfortunate that this programme appeared at such a bad time for you. The people who make these programmes do not realize the fear and anxiety that they can cause.

First you must believe that your son needs insulin – without it he would soon become very ill. It does not really matter at this stage what sort of insulin he has, although most doctors in this country start people who need insulin on the human variety. The only problems with human insulin seem to be caused by the change over from animal to human insulin. As your son has been on human insulin from the start he should not run into any difficulties. Perhaps you should talk to a family in which one of the children has had diabetes for a few years. They would probably be able to give the reassurance you need. You could try the local Diabetes UK voluntary group as a contact. Even if the Parents Group is not attached to Diabetes UK, they should be able to give you a contact number.

I was changed from pork to human insulin 4 years ago and I have not really noticed any difference. I have recently heard that human insulin can be dangerous. Should I be worried?

There has been adverse publicity about human insulin, which has been mentioned in the preceding questions. A number of people changing from animal to human insulin have noticed that they get less warning of hypos. This change of awareness may result from other factors (see the section on **Hypos** later in this chapter) but some people are convinced that the problem was caused by human insulin.

There have also been reports of unexpected deaths in people who have changed to human insulin. These deaths may have been due to hypoglycaemia but this has not been proved. Nor has it been shown that the numbers involved have increased since human insulin was introduced. Diabetes UK has been carrying out research into these vital questions but so far no cause for alarm has been found.

There seem to be a lot of different types of insulin on the market. Can you give me some details?

The range of insulins available can be confusing, although they do fall into four separate groups as we have shown in Table 3.1. Please note that the times of insulin action vary greatly from one person to another and those given here must only be regarded as a rough guide.

The vials mentioned in the table are bottles of insulin for use with a syringe, and cartridges are for use with an insulin pen.

I am taking a mixture of short- and intermediate-acting insulin twice a day and do not understand which insulin is working at which time of day.

Many people are confused by the length of action of their insulin particularly when taken more than twice a day. The diagram in Figure 3.1 gives a representation of some commonly used

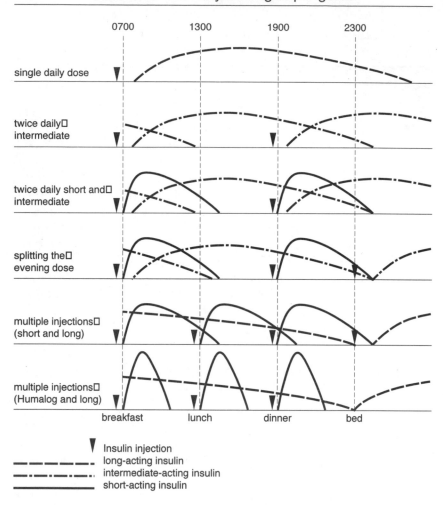

Figure 3.1 Representation of five common insulin regimens.

regimens. However, as a general rule the short-acting insulin works rapidly (morning and evening) and the intermediate-acting insulin takes longer and covers the afternoon and the night. If you are still unclear about it have another word with your doctor or diabetes specialist nurse.

Can I get AIDS from human insulin?

Definitely not. Human insulin is either made from bacteria or yeast 'instructed' to produce insulin that has the same structure as human insulin, or from pork insulin modified to resemble human insulin. It is rigorously purified and cannot be a source of infection.

Is it possible to be allergic to insulin?

Very occasionally people may develop an allergy to one of the additives to insulin such as protamine or zinc, but the insulin itself is unlikely to cause an allergy.

Timing

My doctor is considering changing me from one to two insulin injections per day. Will the second interfere with my social life – eating out, and so on?

No, instead the second injection should make your life more flexible. Most people on one injection a day find that they need a meal in the late afternoon, around 6.00 to 7.00pm. With a second injection, this meal can be delayed for several hours with the insulin given shortly beforehand. With an insulin pen, it is also more convenient to give yourself an insulin injection even when eating out.

I have heard that there is a new fast-acting insulin which is even faster acting than Actrapid. Does it have any advantages?

You are quite right, there are now three new synthetic 'designer' insulins: two rapid-acting insulins – lispro (Humalog) from Lilly, and aspart (NovoRapid) from Novo Nordisk – and two longer-acting versions – glargine (Lantus) from Aventis and detemir

(Levemir) from Novo Nordisk. They are the first of what will be a series of new insulins (known as insulin analogues), which will be produced in the years to come, as we forecast in the last edition of this book. They are designed not to aggregate when injected under the skin (a process that occurs to a varying extent with other insulins), thus facilitating their absorption and action. Their big potential advantage is – at least for Humalog and Novo-Rapid – that they don't need to be injected until immediately before the meal, and their action more closely matches the digestion of the meal than that of conventional clear insulins. This results in better control of the rise in blood glucose following meal digestion and absorption with lowering of the peak glucose concentration. They have another advantage stemming from their short action: when injected before breakfast, they are less likely to cause hypos before lunch as their effects wear off more quickly.

They are ideally suited for the popular 'basal + bolus' regimens (i.e. long acting 'basal' insulin at night with a 'bolus' of short-acting insulin before each meal) and are available in vials, cartridges and disposable pens.

What should I do if I suddenly realize I have missed an injection?

It is quite easy to forget to give yourself an injection or – even worse – to be unable to remember whether or not you have had your injection. If this happens you should measure your blood glucose level to help you decide what to do next.

If your blood glucose is high (more than 10 mmol/litre) you probably did forget your injection and you should have some short-acting insulin as soon as possible. The dose depends on how close you are to the next injection time.

If your blood glucose is normal or low (7 mmol/litre or less) you probably did have your injection even if you have forgotten doing it. It would be safest to check your blood glucose again before your next meal and, if it is high, to have an extra dose of short-acting insulin. Novo Nordisk have recently introduced an insulin doser called Innovo, which has a built-in memory that recalls the amount of dose injected and the number of hours that have elapsed since the last injection.

Does the timing of the injections matter? Can a person who is on two injections a day take them at 10.00am and 4.00pm?

Unless you are taking Humalog or NovoRapid, which are very quick-acting insulins and should be taken just before a meal, it is best to have your insulin about 30 minutes before a meal, and we discuss this further in the next section on *Diet and insulin*. If you have your main meals in the middle of the morning and in the afternoon, then you could try giving insulin at the times you suggest. You may find that an afternoon injection may not last the 18 hours until the next morning – that is why most people try to keep their two injections approximately 12 hours apart.

Dosage

When I was first diagnosed I was put on insulin, but now the dosage has been decreased. The doctor tells me I am in the 'honeymoon period' of diabetes. What does this mean?

People often need a reduction in their insulin dose soon after they start taking insulin for diabetes. This is due to partial recovery of the insulin-producing cells of the pancreas. During this period hypos are often a problem but on the whole it is easy to control the blood glucose during this 'honeymoon'. The honeymoon period usually comes to a sudden end within a few months to a year, often when the person has a bad cold or suffers some other stress to the insulin-producing cells. However, the honeymoon period is a good thing and will improve your chances of successful long-term control of your diabetes.

When I developed diabetes I was started on insulin but kept having hypos, and 3 months ago I came off insulin. Why was I given it in the first place?

Presumably you were given insulin because your doctors thought you needed it. Most people under 40 years old who have ketones in their urine (see the section on *Urine testing* in Chapter 4) are likely to need insulin and tend to be started on this without any delay. When insulin has been given for a week or so, it is quite common for people to be troubled by hypos, in which case the insulin has to be reduced. Sometimes even tiny doses of insulin cause hypos during this 'honeymoon period' (see the previous question) and the injections have to be stopped completely. The honeymoon period may occasionally last as long as a year.

I have had diabetes for 9 months and attend the diabetes clinic every month to have my insulin dose adjusted. How long does it usually take before doctors get you balanced?

This is an interesting question as it assumes that it is up to the doctors to balance your diabetes. Of course the doctors and nurses in the clinic must provide you with all the help and information that you need but, in the end, it is your diabetes for you to control. Good control depends not just on the dose of insulin but the site you choose for your injections, the timing and type of food that you eat and the amount of exercise you take. These are things over which your doctor has no direct control. Most people begin to get their blood glucose under control in a few weeks.

Is my insulin requirement likely to vary at different times of the year because of the weather?

Several people have remarked that their dose of insulin needs to be altered in very hot weather – some need to give themselves more insulin and others less. This is probably because people react in different ways to a heat wave. There is a tendency to eat less and take less exercise in tropical conditions. However, because blood flow to the skin is increased in warm temperatures, this could speed up the absorption of the injected insulin and mean that a given dose will not last as long. Everyone is different and you will have to be on the look out for yourself how hot weather affects your own blood glucose.

If my insulin requirements decrease over the years, does this mean that the pancreas has gradually started to produce more natural insulin than when I was younger?

No. It is most unlikely that after many years of diabetes your pancreas will start to produce natural insulin. However, this reduction in dose in older people is well recognized. It could be that you were having more insulin than you really needed in the past. Since the introduction of blood glucose measurement many people are found to be having too much insulin – or sometimes too much at one time of the day and not enough at another. Other possible explanations for older people needing less insulin are that they eat less food, they become thinner, they have a different exercise pattern, and there may be hormonal changes.

Injecting

Technique

Is it necessary to use spirit before or after injecting myself?

We do not advise you to use spirit or alcohol for cleaning your skin as it is not necessary and it tends to harden the skin. If you feel you must clean the injection site (say after playing football), use soap and water only.

Is it dangerous to inject air bubbles that may be in the syringe after drawing up insulin?

The only reason you are taught to get rid of air bubbles from the syringe after drawing up insulin is because the air takes the place of the insulin and your insulin dose will therefore not be accurate. Very large quantities of air injected directly into the blood circulation could be dangerous and produce an airlock in the bloodstream, but these amounts are far larger than could possibly be introduced when injecting insulin. Moreover, insulin is intended to be injected into the subcutaneous tissue and not into a vein. Tiny air bubbles would not do any harm and would quickly be absorbed, even when introduced into a vein.

Can two types of insulin be mixed in the same syringe?

Yes, many people these days are taking mixtures of insulin. Unless instructed otherwise by your doctor, you should inject mixtures of insulin immediately after they are drawn up, particularly if you are using a zinc-based insulin such as Monotard, Ultratard, Humulin Lente or ZN, Hypurin Lente or PZI.

The rule for mixing insulins is to draw up the clear (short-acting) insulin before the cloudy (intermediate or long-acting) insulin so as to prevent the clear bottle of insulin becoming 'contaminated' by the cloudy insulin. If this happens the clear (short-acting) insulin will lose its quick-acting properties.

When drawing up my insulin I sometimes find that the insulin gets 'sucked back' into the bottle. Why is this?

This is due to a vacuum developing in the vial. It can be easily overcome by injecting a little air into the bottle before drawing the insulin out. Prior to drawing up their insulin, many people routinely put the same amount of air into the bottle as the amount of insulin they intend to draw out to avoid this problem. Research has shown that it may not be necessary to inject air into the bottle, but it is a simple procedure that can prevent the situation you experienced.

I have been giving my insulin injections at an angle of about 45 degrees for many years but have been told that this is incorrect. What do you advise?

Insulin is designed to be injected into the deep layer of fat under the skin – also called subcutaneous tissue – and not into the muscle. In the past, when longer needles were in use, people injecting insulin were taught to lift up their skin and then inject at an angle of 45 degrees. With the introduction of shorter 8 mm needles, teaching gradually changed, and many people learnt to give their injections at right angles to the skin without lifting a skin fold. Recent studies, however, have suggested that, in thin people using this perpendicular injection technique, shorter needles still risk going through the subcutaneous tissue and into the muscle, leading to an erratic and unpredictable absorption of insulin.

The current advice is to give an injection by first lifting up a generous amount of skin (do not squeeze too tightly as this may cause bruising), and then pushing the needle in quickly at right angles to the skin. If the needle is pushed through the skin quickly the injection should be virtually painless.

My young daughter spends a very long time giving her injection and complains that it is painful. Is there any advice you can give?

One of the reasons that she finds it painful is because she is probably pushing the needle slowly through the skin. The sensitive nerve endings lie virtually on the surface of the skin and are more likely to be stimulated if the needle enters the skin very slowly. Try to encourage her to push the needle through the skin as quickly as possible. The use of BD Micro-Fine + needles will also make things easier, particularly if she is using the 5 mm needles. If she still experiences difficulty, then the ice cube technique may be helpful. She can hold a cube of ice against her skin for about 10 seconds – this 'freezes' the skin just long enough for the injection to be given. This method can be used until she has gained more confidence in giving herself her injections.

Sometimes after giving my injection I find that a small lump appears just under the skin. What is the cause of this?

It sounds as though you are giving your injection at too shallow a depth. If the insulin is injected into the skin (intradermally) a small lump will generally appear. Apart from causing more pain, the insulin may not be absorbed properly. Try giving your injection more deeply by injecting at right angles to the skin possibly without a lifted skin fold and this should not happen again.

Should I draw back on the plunger after inserting the needle to check for blood?

It used to be common practice to teach people to draw back on the plunger before injecting insulin to check that the needle had not entered a blood vessel. These days this is not usually taught as the chances of insulin entering a blood vessel are extremely slight, and pulling back the plunger could make the injection more difficult for some people. Moreover, an increasing number of people are now using insulin pens and are unable to 'draw back'. If you are in the habit of drawing back before giving insulin, by all means continue, but it is not strictly necessary.

Sometimes after giving my injection I notice that the injection site bleeds a lot. Does this do any harm?

This may happen if you puncture a blood capillary (a very small blood vessel) which means that the needle goes straight through the capillary. You may then bleed from the injection site and probably see a bruise the following day, but it does no harm. It helps to press quickly with your finger or a tissue over the site. Occasionally this might lead to a slightly faster absorption of insulin.

When I have given my injection I sometimes see some insulin leaking out from the injection hole after taking out the needle. Should I give myself extra insulin later and how much should I give?

Insulin does sometimes leak out immediately after an injection. This can often be avoided by holding the needle in the skin for about 10 seconds allowing then the last drops of insulin to be fully absorbed. An additional precaution could be taken by moving the skin to one side immediately after withdrawing the needle or, alternatively, moving the skin to one side before inserting the needle. This effectively means that the needle channel closes after the needle has been withdrawn. If either of these methods fails then have a tissue handy at injection time ready to press straight on the spot after giving the injection. Extra insulin should not be given if you lose a little because you will not know how much has been lost and will probably overcompensate and risk hypoglycaemia. Having not taken your full dose of insulin may mean that your blood glucose levels might be slightly higher than normal that day.

Sites

Where is the best place to give an injection of insulin?

Insulin is intended to be injected into the deep layers of fat below the skin – also called subcutaneous tissue – and basically can be given in any place where there is a reasonable layer of fat. However, the recommended sites for the injection of insulin are the side of the upper part of thighs, the abdomen at about a hand's breadth to either side of the umbilicus (navel), the upper and lateral part of the arm and the upper outer parts of the buttocks. Some women prefer not to use the arms in the summer months in case they have marks at the injection sites that may be noticeable when they wear summer dresses. It is very important not to develop 'favourite' injection areas, and to change to new sites regularly. Suitable sites for injection are shown in Figure 3.2.

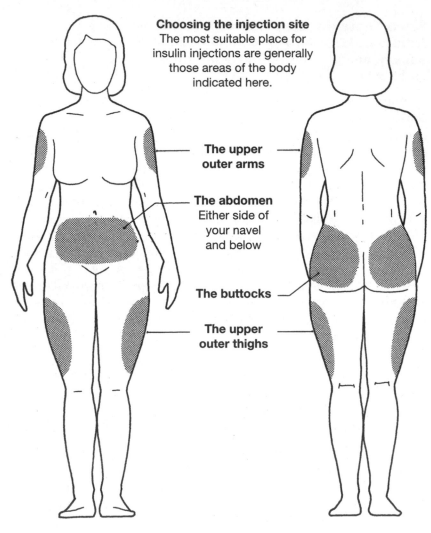

Choosing the injection site
The most suitable place for insulin injections are generally those areas of the body indicated here.

The upper outer arms

The abdomen
Either side of your navel and below

The buttocks

The upper outer thighs

Important
Do not give injections in the same small area.
This may lead to lumpiness of the skin.

Figure 3.2 Injection sites.

I have unsightly lumps on my thighs where I inject my insulin. Could I have plastic surgery to make my thighs smooth again?

If you inject your insulin into the same area every time there is a strong chance that these lumps – also called lipohypertrophy or lipodystrophy – will appear. Some people have similar lumps on their abdomen from repeated injections into the same spot. If you carefully avoid the lumps and inject insulin somewhere else, then the lumps will eventually disappear, although this may take a long time. Apart from looking odd, these lumps can cause your insulin to be absorbed erratically, altering your glycaemic control.

So you can see that it is worth changing to new sites for your injections – the sites you can use are shown in Figure 3.2 – as well as rotating within a given site so as to make sure that you do not inject in the same place as last time. Sometimes it can be difficult to persuade people to change sites to avoid the lumps, as injecting into them is less painful. Unfortunately, they will only tend to get larger if you keep using them. Plastic surgery would leave a scar and is not recommended, although liposuction has had varying degrees of success.

The layer of fat beneath the surface of the skin of my thighs is very hard and I find it difficult to inject myself. Have you any suggestions?

This could be because you are not rotating injection sites and are reusing the same place too many times. This causes your flesh to become hard and the absorption of the insulin to be erratic. These over-used areas should not be injected for about a year and new areas should be found instead (you will find suggestions for suitable sites in Figure 3.2).

Another possible cause for hard skin is the use of spirit for swabbing the skin. This is unnecessary and makes the skin tough and difficult to inject. Stop swabbing your skin and try softening it by rubbing in hand cream at night.

I have been taking insulin for 18 years and have unsightly bulges at the top of my thighs where I give my injections. How can I get rid of them?

These bulges, also known as lipohypertrophy, are a build-up of fat below the skin related to the injection of insulin. This is almost certainly caused by your constantly injecting insulin into the same site over several years. Insulin will not be absorbed properly from these areas and you should not use these sites again for at least a year. Instead inject into your abdomen, buttocks and upper arms until your thighs have been 'rested'. When you return to using your thighs, use a much larger area than before, and try to avoid the top of the thigh.

I have to increase my dose of insulin by four units when injecting into my arms and by 6 units when injecting into the abdomen to maintain control. Can you tell me why this is, and should I inject only into my thighs?

It is known that insulin is absorbed at different rates from different areas of the body. The fastest rate of absorption is from the abdomen and arms, and the slowest from the thighs and buttocks. For many people this will not make much difference to their control, but for others the difference may be significant, and you may be one of these people. You may wish to see if injecting into different areas affects your control by taking several blood glucose measurements at different times of the day each time you choose a new area.

Insulin is also more quickly absorbed from the thighs and buttocks if exercise is taken immediately after the injection. Heat also influences the rate of absorption of insulin, and it will be more quickly absorbed following a hot bath, after sunbathing in a hot country or after using a sun bed.

After using the tops of my thighs for my injection for many years I have recently started using my abdomen but now seem to have hypos every day. Why is this?

This is probably due to insulin being poorly absorbed in the past from your much-used injection areas. We normally suggest that people reduce their dose of insulin when changing to a new or rarely used area because the insulin is usually more effectively absorbed from these new areas, particularly if the dose has slowly increased over the years owing to the injection being given in the same place continually.

Insulin pens

What is an insulin pen, and what are the advantages of using one?

An insulin pen consists of a cartridge of insulin inside a fountain pen type case which is used with a special disposable needle. After dialling the required number of units of insulin you need and inserting the needle into the skin, you press a button and the pen will release the correct dose of insulin.

Several makes of pen are available and your specialist nurse or doctor will show you the current models. They may be used with any of the cartridges listed in Table 3.1. Novopens are supplied by Novo Nordisk, HumaPen by Eli Lilly, OptiPen by Aventis Pharma and Autopens by Owen Mumford (Medical Shop). Insulin pens are now available on prescription except for the Humapen and the Optipen. They should be available free of charge from your diabetes clinic. There is a list of available insulin pens in Table 3.2. Addresses of manufacturers are listed in Appendix 3.

Insulin cartridges and the pen needles for all these pens can be prescribed by your doctor.

Preloaded pens, also called disposable pens, which contain 300 units of insulin, are obtainable on prescription. They are available with most or part of NovoNordisk, Eli Lilly and Aventis Pharma insulin range. The preloaded pens are listed in Table 3.1.

Table 3.2 Insulin pens

Company	Pen name	Dosage	Cartridge size min–max	Insulin used in pen
Owen Mumford	Autopen	1–16 units	150 units (1.5ml)	all types of 1.5ml cartridges
	Autopen 1.5 ml	2–32 units	150 units (1.5ml)	all types of 1.5ml cartridges
	Autopen 3.0 ml	2–42 units	300 units (3ml)	all types of 3ml cartridges except Novo Nordisk 3ml
Novo Nordisk	Novopen 3 Classic	1–70 units	300 units (3ml)	Novo Nordisk Penfill 3ml cartridge
	Novopen 3 Demi	0.5–35 units	300 units (3ml)	Novo Nordisk Penfill 3ml cartridge
	Novopen 3 Fun Junior	1–35 units	300 units (3ml)	Novo Nordisk Penfill 3ml cartridge
	Preloaded pens	2–78 units	300 units (3ml)	Novo Nordisk Penfill 3ml prefilled insulin
	FlexPen	1–60 units	300 units (3ml)	Novo Nordisk 3ml prefilled insulin
	PenMate (hides needle)			Novo Nordisk Penfill 3ml cartridge
	Innovo (with memory)	1–70 units	300 units (3ml)	Novo Nordisk Penfill 3ml cartridge
	InnoLet (for elderly)	1–50 units	300 units (3ml)	Novo Nordisk 3ml prefilled insulin
Lilly	Humapen Ergo 3	1–60 units	300 units (3ml)	Lilly Humulin cartridges
	Humaject prefilled pen	2–96 units	300 units (3ml)	Lilly prefilled insulin
	Humalog Mix 25 pen	1–60 units	300 units (3ml)	Lilly Humalog Mix 25
Aventis Pharma	OptiPen Pro 1	1–60 units	300 units (3ml)	Insuman cartridges
	Aventis Optiset	2–40 units	300 units (3ml)	Insuman prefilled insulin

People wishing to continue to use animal insulin in a pen can do so by using Hypurin neutral, Hypurin isophane or Hypurin 30/70 mix cartridges manufactured by CP Pharmaceuticals. These cartridges are recommended for use with the Owen Mumford Autopen.

The great advantage of insulin pens is convenience and ease of use. It is simple to give an injection away from home, e.g. in a restaurant or when travelling. If you are visually impaired, or if you suffer from arthritis in your hands, then you may find the dial-a-dose clicking action is easier to use than drawing up insulin in a conventional syringe.

All these pens rely on ordinary finger pressure for the injection, i.e. they are not automatic injectors.

If you are afraid of needles, finding it difficult to inject your insulin but still would like to use a pen, Novo Nordisk have introduced the Penmate which hides the needle from view when the injection is given. Addresses for all the companies mentioned in this answer can be found in Appendix 3.

What is the advantage of taking four injections a day with an insulin pen?

The idea of using a multiple injection regimen is to try to mimic the normal secretion of the pancreas by giving small doses of short-acting insulin to cover meals and a longer-acting insulin at bedtime to act as a background insulin. This system should really be called basal + bolus, i.e. long acting 'basal' insulin at night with a 'bolus' of short-acting insulin before each meal. It is more convenient to implement with the use of an insulin pen.

Some people who lead rather erratic lives find the insulin pen regimen more convenient. They have a little more flexibility over the timing of their meals, as the insulin is not taken until just before the meal is eaten. In practice they may also need some longer-acting insulin taken in the morning to act as a background insulin. Another advantage of using an insulin pen is that bottles of insulin do not need to be carried around during the day, and it is easier to give an injection discreetly.

Pumps and injectors

I have heard about insulin pumps for treating diabetes. Doctors in my own clinic never seem very keen on the idea. How do pumps work and are they a good form of treatment?

First, an explanation of why insulin pumps have been developed. People who do not have diabetes release a very small amount of insulin into the bloodstream throughout the day and over the night. This insulin prevents the liver from releasing its glucose stock into the bloodstream. Whenever the glucose level rises after a meal the pancreas immediately produces extra insulin to damp the level down. This is a simple feedback system designed to keep the level of blood glucose steady. Without the 'background' insulin in between meals, the level of blood glucose would slowly rise.

Insulin pumps are an attempt to copy this normal pattern. They consist of a slow motor driving a syringe or cartridge containing insulin, which is pumped down a fine-bore tube and needle. The needle is inserted under the skin and strapped in place. There is also a device for giving mealtime boosts of insulin. The modern pumps are about the size of a pager, and a microprocessor-based button allows a wide range of rate settings.

Many people have successfully controlled their blood glucose with an insulin pump. However, they are not curently available on the NHS, and they are very expensive to buy and run. They require extra blood tests and adjustments in the dose of insulin, but they can be a good way of achieving tight control of diabetes in people with a high degree of commitment. Since the introduction of insulin pens, pumps became less popular, but they are gaining favour in some centres.

My diabetes is well controlled. Should I be thinking of buying a pump?

Probably not, if your diabetes really is well controlled. Pumps are only used in a small number of diabetes clinics throughout the UK, although their use is becoming more widespread.

Currently approximately 0.1% of people with Type 1 diabetes in the UK use pumps, compared with about 5% in the USA, the Netherlands, Sweden, Germany and Norway. Pump therapy is not suitable for all people with diabetes. From discussions with healthcare professionals, pump users and manufacturers, the people most suited to using pumps must be well motivated and willing to take control of their diabetes, have a good knowledge and understanding of their diabetes, and be prepared to test blood glucose levels at least four times a day and be able to act on those results.

NICE (National Institute for Clinical Excellence), a government body which assesses the value of new forms of treatment, has reviewed the clinical and cost effectiveness of insulin pump therapy. They will report their findings soon. They may recommend that, under certain circumstances, pumps should be funded by the NHS – this would provide a welcome boost to this method of giving insulin.

Research has shown that, if you are the sort of person who achieves good control by giving insulin with modern insulin regimens, then you would probably be able to do slightly better using a pump but, if your control is normally erratic, then equipping you with a pump is not likely to improve matters.

What are the main difficulties of using a pump for giving insulin?

The main problem with pumps is that, like all machines, they are capable of going wrong. One reason for the high cost of insulin pumps is the need to build a warning system into the design to alert the user to a mechanical fault. If the pump suddenly stops, the user will rapidly go into a state of complete insulin lack and may quickly develop ketoacidosis.

Also, because the needle remains under the skin it acts as a foreign body and may set up a focus of infection leading to an abscess. The needle must be inserted only after careful cleaning of the skin and must be replaced every 2 days.

From the user's point of view, the main disadvantage of the pump is the fact that it has to be worn day and night. This is obviously less convenient than the ordinary injections, which are over and done with. Many people dislike the pump because they find it to be a constant reminder of their diabetes.

How can I obtain an insulin pump?

The first thing to do is to discuss the use of the pump with your diabetes specialist. If they feel that you are a suitable candidate, but they have little experience with pumps themselves, they may need to refer you to another centre. Pumps are not currently available on the NHS, and at the moment (see previous questions) UK funding for pump treatment is met by a mixture of local charities, purchase by people with diabetes themselves, research trials and private donations to hospitals. At the time of writing there are two manufacturers supplying pumps in the UK. The Disetronic H-Tron pump has a programmed 2 year lifetime. The Minimed model 505 has a single basal rate, and the model 507 has multiple basal rates. Minimed pumps and supplies can be obtained from their distributor, Applied Medical Technology. These pumps are estimated to have a lifetime of 7 years. All pumps are very expensive to buy and they have weekly running costs. Both Disetronic and Applied Medical Technology have nurse educators who will initiate pump treatment either at the diabetes centre or in the home. Both AMT and Disetronic state that they will only supply pumps and instruct people with the close cooperation of the doctor managing the client's diabetes (addresses in Appendix 3). Diabetes UK will have details on pumps as well.

Injectors

My son has trouble giving himself injections and has asked me if he can use an injector. What type of injector should he use?

With insulin pens and thin diameter disposable needles injections are rarely a problem if the correct technique is used. Most people find injectors more trouble than they are worth, and they are something extra to carry around, but they may help people like your son who are going through a difficult patch.

Injectors work on a similar principle of pushing the needle very quickly through the skin, whilst hiding the needle from view. As well as offering fast needle penetration, the Auto-Injector also automatically delivers the insulin at speed with a conventional syringe. Its disadvantages are that it is rather noisy and over-sized. It is obtainable from Owen Mumford (Medical Shop) (address in Appendix 3). This injector is not available on pre-scription. If your son uses an insulin pen, Novo Nordisk have introduced a device called PenMate, which slips over the NovoPen 3 and inserts the needle into the skin automatically, whilst hiding it from view.

What is the 'jet' injector?

This is a needle-free injector, which works by firing liquid, such as insulin, through the skin from very high pressure jets. It is not entirely painless, is bulky, expensive, not available on the NHS, and has not yet been proved to be harmless when multiple injec-tions are given. As with needles, potential problems of bruising can occur. These injectors are no longer marketed in the UK, but can be obtained from suppliers in the USA. Diabetes UK can sup-ply these addresses, but like ourselves, they do not recommend their use.

Practical aspects of syringes, needles and bottles

When I was discharged from hospital with newly diagnosed diabetes I was given a few disposable syringes and needles for my injections. How do I obtain more?

Disposable insulin syringes and pen needles are available free on prescription. Your GP will supply you with a prescription for any make of insulin syringe and/or insulin pen needles that you choose and they can then be obtained free from the chemist. Alternatively you can buy them directly from the chemist without a prescription (although you will have to pay for them), or you can send for them by post from suppliers such as Owen Mumford (Medical Shop). Their address is in Appendix 3.

What is the best way of disposing of insulin syringes and needles?

There is a device available called the BD Safe-Clip which cuts the needle off the top of the syringe or insulin pen and retains it in the device. Once the needle is clipped off, put the used syringe or pen needle hub into a rigid sealable container along with your lancets and follow your local council guidelines for safe disposal of medical waste. Some local authorities provide special containers and a collection service for people who are treated with insulin; however, there is no national policy.

The BD Safe-Clip is available free on prescription from your GP.

I have heard that disposable syringes and needles can be reused. How many times can they be reused and how can they be kept clean in between injections?

While disposable syringes and pen needles are designed to be used only once, some people do reuse them. However, reusing needles causes them to become blunt, and they twist and bend. The tiny point on the end can also break off and remain embedded in the subcutaneous tissue. Needles have a fine coating of lubricant on them so they glide in and out of the skin, and reusing them removes this lubricant and may cause a painful injection. So there are many reasons why it is logical to use each needle once only.

If you decide to reuse them, keep the syringe dry and in a clean place with the protective cover placed over the needle.

There is a bewildering array of syringes and needles on the market. Which are the best types to use?

In this country there are three sizes of syringe to be used with U100 insulin (this is the standard strength of insulin in the UK, and most countries, and refers to 100 units of insulin per 1 millilitre):

- the more commonly used, the 0.5 ml syringe, marked with 50 single divisions for those taking not more than 50 units of insulin in one injection;
- the 1 ml syringe, marked up to 100 units in 2 unit divisions for those taking more than 50 units of insulin in one injection; and
- the 0.3 ml syringe, more specifically designed for children or those taking less than 30 units of insulin in one injection.

All these syringes are marked with the word INSULIN on the side of the syringe and graduated in units of insulin. No other

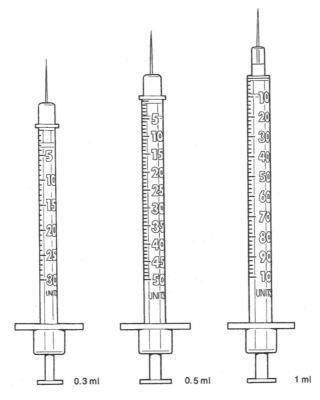

Figure 3.3 Insulin syringes — 0.3 ml, 0.5 ml and 1 ml.

type should be used when an insulin injection is given. They are all shown in Figure 3.3.

Note that one division on the 0.3 ml and 0.5 ml syringes is equal to 1 unit of insulin, while on the 1 ml syringe one division is equal to 2 units of insulin.

The most popular syringe is the BD syringe which comes complete with a fixed Micro-Fine+ 12.7 mm needle, but there are several other makes available.

What length of needle should I use on my insulin pen?

There are several lengths of needle available today ranging from 5 mm to 12.7 mm. The general rule is to use the 5 or 6 mm needle for children and thin to normal weight adults without a lifted skin fold; the 8 mm for normal weight adults with a lifted skin fold, and the 12 or 12.7 mm needle for overweight adults also with a lifted skin fold. Ask your healthcare professional for the needle length and injection technique the most appropriate for you.

I am partially sighted. What syringes are available for people like me, or for people who are blind? Are there any gadgets that would help me with my injections?

Most visually impaired people would be advised to use an insulin pen but, if you wish to use a syringe, BD and Sherwood can supply magnifiers that clip over their plastic syringes, which may make the marks easier to read. An insulin pen is probably the best choice for people like you who are visually impaired. It is quite easy to use once the technique has been mastered, and offers a good choice of insulin regimens. This should be discussed with your physician or diabetes specialist nurse. There is a section about ***Insulin pens*** earlier in this chapter.

Novo Nordisk have recently introduced a device called Innolet that might well suit you. It is a disposable insulin pen with a large clock-like dial, audible clicks accompanying each unit dialled, and which is easy to hold as it has a large grip.

Where should I keep my supplies of insulin?

Stores of insulin should ideally be kept in a refrigerator, but not in the freezer or freezing compartment. The ideal storage temperature is between 2° and 8°C. Below 0°C insulin is destroyed, and from 30°C upwards, insulin activity progressively decreases. If you do not have a fridge, then insulin may be stored for about a month at room temperature but keep it away from direct heat such as radiators and strong sunlight. Many people prefer to keep their insulin bottle and/or their insulin pen in current use at room temperature as it may make the injection more comfortable (cold insulin increases the pain of the injection).

Should I wipe the top of the insulin bottle with spirit before drawing up the required dose?

Although some clinics teach people to clean the tops of the insulin bottles, we do not think that it is necessary.

Diet and insulin

I have been told that I am going to have to start insulin after many years of diet and tablets. Will my diet need to change?

Possibly, and in any case it would be helpful for you to have the opportunity to discuss your present eating habits with your dietitian before you start on insulin. If you have been trying to avoid going on to insulin by restricting the amount of carbohydrate you eat, you may well be advised to increase your intake.

I am quite a thin person but have been told to watch my 'diet'. Why?

The word 'diet' can often be misleading, as many people think of a diet only in terms of a weight-reducing diet. In fact, the word diet just means a way of eating or a prescribed course of food, and for a person with diabetes it simply means planned eating. It might be better if we all used the terms 'food plan' or 'eating plan' instead, but most of us just continue to use the word 'diet' in our everyday conversation!

The reason everyone with diabetes needs a food plan is to help them balance the amount of food that they eat against the amount of insulin and exercise they take. The simplest plan just encourages you to eat some carbohydrate foods at each meal. Carbohydrate foods are starchy or sugary foods such as bread, biscuits, crackers, crispbreads, pasta, potatoes, pulses, cereals, rice, fruit, and so on.

A more detailed plan would tell you about the amounts of proteins and fats that you should eat. Proteins are an essential part of everyone's food intake but are only needed in moderate amounts. Foods high in proteins include meat, fish, eggs, cheese, pulses and nuts. Fats are used for energy and are a more concentrated source of calories than either carbohydrate or protein. However, you should pay attention to the quantity of fat you eat – taken in excess, fat can lead to weight gain and may contribute to heart disease in later life. Examples of fats are butter, cream, margarine, lard and vegetable oils. Fried food, cakes and pastries are also high in fats.

Most people eat roughly the same amount of food each day and so, when you are trying to balance food, insulin and exercise, it makes sense to keep your carbohydrate and calorie intake fairly constant, so that only your insulin and the amount of exercise you take need to be adjusted. The aim of your food plan is to eat roughly the same amounts of carbohydrates and calories at much the same time every day. The dietitian will firstly assess your previous diet and then advise you on the essential changes you need to make whilst trying to retain as much as possible of your previous eating pattern.

**My 16-year-old son has had diabetes since he was 6. We
have managed quite well but since he has been
transferred to the diabetes clinic we have seen more of
the dietitian. I am confused – she spends time urging us to
eat more fibre-rich foods and cut down the fats. He's not
overweight and has never had a problem with his bowels.**

Different foods or meals affect blood glucose levels in varying
ways even when their carbohydrate content is the same. It's the
total number of calories you eat not just the amount of carbohydrates that affects whether or not you are overweight, and a
fibre-rich diet will actually be good for all of you, not just your
bowels.

There is now a lot more emphasis on the type and quality of
the carbohydrate foods we eat. Carbohydrates that are rich in
fibre (those with a low glycaemic index – see the next question)
usually take longer to digest, do not raise the blood glucose quite
so much or so quickly, and keep blood glucose at a steady level
for longer, which helps to prevent hypos. They also contain more
vitamins and minerals and are believed to prevent the build-up of
excess fat in the arteries. The amount of heart disease amongst
people with diabetes (and the general population) worries the
experts and this is why there is much more emphasis on the
whole diet, particularly in eating more of the fibre-rich foods and
cutting back on fatty foods.

**I gather different forms of carbohydrate have different
rates of digestion and that this affects the rise in blood
glucose after a meal. I gather there is a 'glycaemic index'
for each type of carbohydrate. What is this glycaemic
index?**

Yes, you are quite right. Many carbohydrate foods have been
graded according to the extent that they put the blood glucose up
after a given amount. Refined carbohydrate (like sugar) and
some other foodstuffs (e.g. potatoes) have a high glycaemic
index, while some unrefined carbohydrates like rice and pasta
have a much lower index. This means that within your calorie-

controlled diet, you can most likely be able to eat more rice and pasta than sugar and potatoes and still maintain the same level of blood glucose control. Although every person is different, the foodstuffs with a high glycaemic index should be taken sparingly while you will find that you can probably be more liberal with foods with a low glycaemic index without upsetting your glycaemic control. On the other hand you may also be able to improve your control by increasing the proportion of carbohydrates of low glycaemic index in your diet. You need to be aware of the possible need for a reduction in insulin dose under these circumstances. More information on glycaemic index can be found on a website given in Appendix 3 (see also the *Diet* section in Chapter 2).

How long before eating should I have my insulin injection?

People who do not have diabetes start to produce insulin at the very beginning of a meal. Since it takes some time for injected insulin to be absorbed, you should ideally aim to have your insulin injection about 30 minutes before your meal, unless you are taking Humalog or NovoRapid, which should be given just before a meal. If your blood glucose level is low at the time of the injection there should be less delay between your insulin and your food.

I am on two injections a day. Sometimes I find it inconvenient to take my evening injection. Can I skip it and have a meal containing no carbohydrate?

No, you cannot skip your evening injection. When the effect of your morning injection wears out, your blood glucose levels will rise even if you have no carbohydrates to eat. Nowadays you can use an insulin pen, which makes it more convenient to inject insulin.

Do people taking insulin need to eat snacks in between meals?

Sometimes, yes. When your pancreas functions normally, it produces insulin 'on demand' when you eat and 'switches off' when the food has been used up. Injected insulin does not 'switch off' in this way. As injected insulin has a peak effect at certain times of the day, it is important for you to cover its action by eating a certain amount of carbohydrates, or you will have a hypo. It is worth remembering that the carbohydrates will last longer if they are rich in fibre (with a low glycaemic index), as they are then more slowly absorbed.

If you find it difficult to eat between meals it may be possible to cut down the number of snacks that you need by changing from a short-acting insulin to an intermediate-acting insulin, although some people still need to eat snacks even when taking a longer-acting insulin, particularly if they are very active. Alternatively, you could try a new very short-acting insulin analogue. There are many ways in which you can adjust your insulin regimen to suit the life you want to lead, and your doctor or diabetes specialist nurse will be able to advise you about these.

As I have to take insulin should I eat a bedtime snack?

Generally speaking, no, unless your blood glucose level is less than 7 mmol/litre at bedtime. If it is lower than this, or if you have hypos during the night (blood glucose tends to fall during the night) then you might need a bedtime snack. Something like a bowl of cereal, a piece of bread or toast, a sandwich, or some wholemeal crispbreads will last you better through the night than a rapidly absorbed milk or fruit juice drink with biscuits. If you are on insulin, you may do better by adjusting your dose – there is a question about this in the section on *Hypos* later in this chapter.

Should I increase my insulin over Christmas to cope with the extra food I shall be eating?

Yes, you can take extra insulin to cover the extra carbohydrates that you eat on any special occasion, not just Christmas. At Christmas everyone (including people with diabetes) eats more and it is best to accept this – but you also have to accept that extra food will increase your waistline!

Extra food does need extra insulin and it is up to you to try to discover by how many units you should increase your dose. You will probably need to work this out by trial and error, but firstly we would suggest that you do not increase the insulin by more than four units at a time, best taken in a quick-acting form shortly before your meal.

Don't forget the effect of exercise on your blood glucose – the traditional afternoon stroll after Christmas lunch is a good idea.

Is it all right for me, as someone who takes insulin, to have a lie-in on Sunday or must I get up and have my injection and breakfast at the normal time?

As with many of the answers in this book, the best advice we can give is try it and see on a couple of occasions. Try the effect of delaying your morning injection and breakfast and measure your blood glucose when you get up 3 or 4 hours later. If it is well below 10 mmol/litre, all well and good, but if your blood glucose is higher than 10 mmol/litre it means that you should not have missed your insulin. You may have to persuade someone else to give your morning injection and bring you breakfast in bed!

I have two injections a day: morning and evening. I keep regular times for breakfast and evening tea but I would like to vary the time that I take lunch. What effect would this have on the control of my diabetes?

This is a difficult problem for someone on insulin. Because of your morning injection, you may tend to feel hypo if you are late for lunch. If your morning injection is mainly intermediate-acting insulin (e.g. Humulin I, Monotard, Insulatard or Insuman Basal), you may be able to delay your lunch a little provided that you have a mid-morning snack. Have you thought of having multiple injections using an insulin pen? There is a section on *Insulin pens* later in this chapter.

Sometimes I suffer from a poor appetite. Is it all right for me to reduce my insulin dose on such occasions?

Yes, that is perfectly acceptable provided that you do not miss out completely on a main meal. You will have to find out for yourself (by measuring your blood glucose) by how much you should reduce your insulin for a particular amount of food. If you are underweight do not reduce your food intake too drastically. On the other hand, if you are overweight, you will need to reduce both your food intake and your insulin.

My daughter has had diabetes for 4 years and has had no problems with her diet. She takes part in most school sports but, since she has taken up running longer distances, she finds that she has a hypo about 2 hours after she has finished running. She has no problems during the run so what should she do to counteract this?

The effect of exercise on the body can last well after the exercise has stopped, as the muscles are restocking their energy stores with glycogen. Your daughter is obviously taking in enough food to last her during her run, but not enough to keep her going through this 'restocking' process. She would probably find it helpful to eat an extra carbohydrate snack, such as a fruit juice and a sandwich, after her run has finished. It might also be a good idea for her to reduce her morning dose of insulin on the days she is running. We talk more about balancing insulin, food and exercise in the section on *Sports* in Chapter 5.

My son has been putting on weight since being diagnosed as having diabetes 3 months ago. What are the reasons for this?

Most people lose weight before their diabetes is diagnosed and treated. In uncontrolled diabetes body fat is broken down and many calories are lost as glucose in the urine (this is discussed in more detail in the section on *Symptoms* in Chapter 1). As soon as the diabetes is brought under control, the body fat stops being broken down, the calories are no longer lost and the weight loss stops. Many people, like your son, begin to put weight back on again.

If your son starts to put on too much weight, he should discuss this with his diabetes specialist nurse and his dietitian. They will advise him about his diet and, if he is on insulin, about reducing his food intake and his insulin simultaneously.

I have been taking insulin for 8 years and over this time I have put on a lot of weight. My doctor says that insulin does not make you fat, but if that is so, then why have I put on so much weight?

People tend to lose weight if their diabetes is badly controlled, mainly because they are losing a lot of calories as glucose in their urine (this is discussed in more detail in the section on *Symptoms* in Chapter 1). Once the diabetes is controlled, the calories are no longer lost in this way, the weight loss stops, and there will be a tendency for a person starting treatment to put on weight. Insulin in the right dose does not make you fat, but if you are having too much insulin you will have to eat more to prevent hypos, and these extra calories will increase your weight.

When you are on insulin and become overweight, then losing the extra weight can be a slow business. You cannot afford the luxury of sudden, drastic dieting (not that this is recommended for anyone – it is not the best way to lose weight) but can lose weight only by careful reduction of both food and insulin. This can be a delicate balance but many people do manage it successfully.

There is a particular risk of weight gain when children stop growing. Children need enormous amounts of food when they are actually growing taller, but once fully grown they need to make a conscious effort to reduce their total food intake. Girls usually stop growing a year or two after their first period and unless they eat a lot less at that stage they will almost certainly become overweight – and will find that it is much easier to put on weight than to take it off.

Since I went onto multiple injections to improve my control and fit them in with my hectic work schedule I have put on quite a lot of weight. I am really pleased with my control but I know in part it is because I take my insulin now whereas I often didn't before because of the fear of hypos. Why do I keep on getting fatter?

The new system is helping you control your diabetes in your hectic lifestyle but it is important to realize that now you are taking your insulin at the right time all the food you eat is going to be used, and the excess is going to be stored as fat!

To control your weight you need to balance the food you eat with the amount of energy you use up. You should aim for a weight loss of between 0.5–1 kg (1–2 lb) a week. Start by looking at the amounts of fat and alcohol in your diet, as these are both very concentrated sources of calories. Try to cut back on fatty foods, perhaps by having low fat products instead of full fat, and having fruit or a diet yoghurt instead of crisps or biscuits, as snacks. Always choose lean rather than fatty meat or replacing it with fish or poultry with the skin removed. If your weight loss slows up or stops, then be prepared to consider reducing also your intake of starchy foods.

Before you start to notice a drop in weight your control might well improve further, so do be prepared to monitor your blood glucose and reduce your insulin as necessary. Regular exercise will help burn off some of the fat and stop the problem developing in the future. If your weight continues to be a problem, record all your meals and snacks for 3 or 4 days and then ask the dietitian to go over them with you to see where further changes can be made.

My 18-year-old daughter has diabetes and is trying to lose weight. She eats a low-carbohydrate diet and sticks to this rigidly. I cannot understand why she does not lose any weight.

Just reducing the amount of carbohydrate in her diet will not necessarily result in her losing weight. When you are trying to lose weight it is important to reduce the total number of calories in your diet, and this involves reducing the amounts of fat, protein, and alcohol you consume – particularly fat as it is such a concentrated form of calories. Your daughter should avoid fried foods, sugary foods and alcohol, cut down her cheese intake, substitute skimmed milk for ordinary full-fat milk and allow only a scraping of butter or margarine on her bread. She will find a diet that contains plenty of high-fibre carbohydrates will be more satisfying and cause less fluctuation in her blood glucose and, as a result, it will be easier for her to follow. Ask your daughter to seek help from her doctor, dietitian and diabetes specialist nurse so that they can work together to prevent hypoglycaemia.

Hypos

Since my wife has been started on insulin she has had funny turns. What is the cause of this?

Your wife's funny turns are likely to be due to a low blood glucose level. The medical term is hypoglycaemia that most people call 'hypo' for short.

When the blood glucose level falls below a certain level (usually 3 mmol/litre), the brain is affected. Highly dependent on glucose, the brain stops working properly and begins to produce symptoms such as weakness of the legs, double or blurred vision, confusion, headache and, in severe cases, loss of consciousness and convulsions. Hypoglycaemia will also trigger the production of adrenaline, an hormone that will be responsible for causing sweating, rapid heartbeat and feelings of panic and anxiety.

Table 3.3 Symptoms of hypo in groups

Cause	Symptom
Due to adrenaline response	Sweating Pounding heart Shaking/trembling Hunger Anxiousness Tingling
Due to brain lack of glucose	Confusion/difficulty in thinking Drowsiness/weakness Odd (stroppy) behaviour Speech difficulty
Non-specific	Nausea Headache Tiredness

Children often describe a 'dizzy feeling' or just 'tiredness' when they are hypo. Most people find it hard to describe how they feel when hypo but the proof is that the blood glucose is low. If there is any doubt about the accuracy of your meter readings, it is always safer to take glucose or sugar if you're feeling odd. A list of hypo symptoms is given in Table 3.3.

What is the best thing to take when I have a hypo?

This very much depends at which stage you recognize the hypo is developing. In the early stages the best treatment would be to have a meal or snack if one is due; or an extra snack such as a fruit, sandwich or biscuits if there is some time before your next meal.

If your hypo is fairly well advanced then you need to take some very rapidly absorbed carbohydrates. This is best taken as sugar, sweets or fruit juice or, for even greater speed, a sugary drink such as ordinary (not 'diet') Coke, lemonade or Lucozade. Good things to carry in your pocket are also glucose tablets such as Dextro-Energy as they are absorbed very quickly (three tablets of

Dextro-Energy contain 10 g of glucose). They are also less likely to be eaten when you are not hypo than ordinary sweets!

Do not forget to eat some bread, biscuits or a small sandwich after the sugar or sugary drink!

I am taking soluble and isophane insulin twice a day and am getting hypos 2 to 3 hours after my evening meal. As I live alone this has been worrying me. What can I do?

Anyone who is having frequent hypos at a particular time of day can easily put this right by adjusting their insulin dose. In this case, you are having hypos at the time when your evening dose of soluble insulin is working. You should reduce the amount of soluble insulin you take in the evening until you have stopped having hypos at that time. On the other hand, hypos before your evening meal could be corrected by reducing your morning dose of inter-mediate-acting (isophane) insulin.

My teenage daughter has diabetes and sometimes turns very nasty and short-tempered. Is this due to the insulin?

Yes, probably – although it is not the only cause of bad moods in teenagers! The only way to find out is to try to persuade her to have a blood glucose measurement during her bad moods. If it is low (3 mmol/litre or less) she is then experiencing a hypo and some glucose should restore her good nature. Because the brain is affected by a low blood glucose level, irrational behaviour is common during a hypo. Your daughter may forcibly deny that she is hypo and resist taking the glucose her body needs. If you are firm and do not panic you will be able to talk her into taking the glucose (Lucozade, lemonade or Coke can be useful here) and she will soon be back to normal.

Children and adults can also become irritable if their blood glucose is very high.

My 8-year-old son often complains of feeling tired after recovering from a hypo. Is this usual and what is the best way to overcome it?

It is unusual to feel tired for more than 30 minutes after a hypo but, if your son does so, you should first check his blood glucose. If this is more than 4 mmol/litre you will just have to let him rest until he is back to normal. It is not uncommon for hypos to trigger headaches and migraine attacks, which may be the problem here.

My teenage son refuses to take extra carbohydrate when he is hypo and insists that we let him sleep it off. Is this all right?

Hypos should always be corrected as quickly as possible. Your son is right in thinking that the insulin will eventually wear off and that his blood glucose will return to normal. However, if his blood glucose falls to very low levels, it could cause problems and he may even become unconscious. His refusal to take sugar is part of the confusion that occurs during a hypo and, if he can be persuaded to take glucose, he will get better more quickly.

I have been taking insulin for 38 years and my hypos have always been mild. Recently I suffered two blackouts lasting a minute, which I presume were hypos. Why has this started?

Blackouts tend to occur in children who have not yet learned to recognize the warning signs of a hypo but, on rare occasions, anyone on insulin can be caught unawares and have a sudden hypo, which makes them black out.

Sometimes as people get older the 'adrenaline' warnings of a hypo fail to operate. This failure may be due to the natural ageing process or to damage (caused by diabetes) of the involuntary nerve supply which transmits the warning signs. Recent studies have suggested that keeping blood glucose levels above 4 mmol/litre can help to restore lost hypo warnings. 'Make 4 the floor' is the advice given.

A number of people have also reported that after changing to human insulin they have less warning of hypos. So far there is no explanation for this. We have discussed human insulin in the section on *Types of insulin* at the beginning of this chapter.

I have recently lost my warning signs for hypos. Is it likely that they will return?

Very tight diabetic control is known to reduce hypoglycaemic awareness. In a study carried out with the help of people who had lost their warning symptoms, the results showed that when they ran their blood glucose control so as to prevent low glucose levels altogether for 3 months, partial or complete restoration of warning symptoms was experienced by everyone who had managed to avoid dropping to blood glucose levels of 4 mmol/litre or less. Do you think that you may fall into this category? If so, it may be worth discussing this with your diabetes team and reducing your dose of insulin.

My father has had diabetes for 20 years. Recently he had what his doctor calls epileptic fits. Would you tell me how to help him and if there is a cure?

A bad hypo may bring on a fit and it is important to check your father's blood glucose during an attack. If the glucose level is low then reducing his insulin should stop the fits. If the fits are not due to a low blood glucose level, it should be possible to control them by making sure he takes his tablets regularly – ask his doctor for more details about these.

Can insulin reactions eventually cause permanent brain damage?

This question is often asked and is a great source of anxiety to many people. The brain quickly recovers from a hypo and there is unlikely to be permanent damage, even after a severe attack with convulsions. Very prolonged hypoglycaemia can occur in someone with a tumour that produces insulin, and if someone is unconscious for days on end then the brain will not recover completely. This is not likely to occur in people with diabetes, in whom the insulin wears off after a few hours.

I have heard that there is an opposite to insulin called glucagon. Is this something like glucose and can it be used to bring someone round from a hypo?

Glucagon is a hormone which, like insulin, is produced by the pancreas. It causes glucose to be released into the bloodstream from stores of starch in the liver. Glucagon can also be injected to bring someone round from a hypo if they are too restless to swallow glucose, or unconscious. Glucagon cannot be stored in solution like insulin. It comes in a kit containing a vial with glucagon powder plus a syringe and sterile fluid for dissolving the powder. The process of dissolving the glucagon and drawing it into the syringe may be difficult especially if you are feeling panicky. It is worth asking the diabetes specialist nurse to show you and your likely helper how to draw up glucagon.

It is usually stated that glucagon only has a short-lasting effect and it is therefore important to follow it up with some sugar by mouth to prevent a relapse of coma. However, in children the blood glucose level may rise very high after an injection of glucagon and, as they often feel sick, it seems silly to force more sugar down them. It is best to do a blood test to help decide whether more glucose is really needed immediately. More sustaining carbohydrates (such as bread or biscuits) should be given as soon as they feel well enough to eat, as the blood glucose level can fall again later.

When I gave my wife a glucagon injection recently, she vomited. Is this normal?

Some people do vomit when regaining consciousness after a glucagon injection, particularly children. If only half the content of the vial is given (0.5 mg), it will usually be enough to correct the hypo, but less likely to cause sickness.

**My diabetes was controlled by tablets for 20 years but
2 years ago my doctor recommended that I begin insulin
treatment. I am well controlled but my sleep is often
disturbed by dreams, or I wake up feeling hungry. Can
you advise me what to do if this happens?**

You may be going hypo in the middle of the night. It has been
shown that many people have low blood glucose in the early
hours of the night and, provided that they feel all right and sleep
well, this probably does not matter. However, if you are regularly
waking up with hypo symptoms (such as hunger) or having night-
mares, you should first check whether you are hypo by measuring
your blood glucose level at around 3.00am when your blood
glucose is usually the lowest. If the reading is below 4 mmol/litre
you need to reduce your evening dose of intermediate-acting
insulin. If your blood glucose is then high before breakfast the
next day, an injection of intermediate-acting insulin taken before
going to bed instead of before your evening meal may solve your
problem.

**What can I do if my son has a bad hypo and is too drowsy
to take any glucose by mouth?**

You should try giving him Hypostop. This is a jelly loaded with
glucose, which comes in a container with a nozzle. It can be
squirted onto the gums of someone who is severely hypo and
often leads to recovery within a few minutes. Hypostop is
available on prescription from your GP, or can be obtained from
Bio Diagnostics Ltd (the address is in Appendix 3). If Hypostop
fails, you should try injecting your son with glucagon – there are
some questions about glucagon above.

**Am I correct in thinking that only people on insulin can
have hypos?**

No. Some of the tablets used for treating Type 2 diabetes can also
cause hypos. The commonly used ones are glibenclamide
(Euglucon, Daonil) and gliclazide (Diamicron). These hypos will

improve with glucose in the normal way but, because the tablets have a longer action than insulin, the hypo may return again after several hours. Anyone having hypos on tablets probably needs to reduce the dose. Metformin and the glitazones, however, do not cause hypos.

My diabetes is treated by diet alone and I have headaches and a light-headed feeling around midday if I have been busy in the morning. I am all right after eating something. Why is this?

It seems surprising but some people on diet alone can go hypo if they go without food. This is because they produce their own insulin, but too late and sometimes too much. Ideally you should try to arrange a blood glucose measurement at a time that you feel odd in order to prove that you are actually hypo. If so, you could avoid the problem by eating little and often, especially on days when you are busy.

My daughter aged 21 takes insulin for her diabetes and is moving down to London where she hopes to rent a flat on her own. In view of the risk of hypoglycaemic attacks, would you advise against this?

By the age of 21 your daughter will be ready to be independent and live in a flat by herself. All parents worry when their children leave home, and diabetes adds to their anxiety, but sooner or later young people have to lead separate lives. We know that night hypos are common and that people either wake up and sort themselves out or else their blood glucose returns to normal as the insulin wears off and they wake up next morning unaware of any problem. However, there has been a handful of cases when people on insulin are found unexpectedly dead in bed, and possibly some of these cases are due to hypoglycaemia. This must be a cause of concern but considering the hundreds of thousands of people on insulin, the risk of this tragedy is equivalent to being struck by lightning and young people on insulin have a right to independence.

Your daughter should be aware of the risk of hypo when driving or swimming and be encouraged to tell her close friends and companions about diabetes. They should be told that, if she ever behaves oddly, she must be given some form of sugar, even if she protests. People often fail to take this simple precaution; it can avoid a lot of worry to their friends who may find them hypo and yet have no idea how to help.

4
Monitoring and control

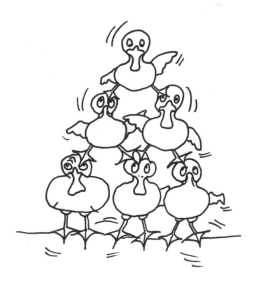

The key to a successful life with diabetes is achieving good blood glucose control. Your degree of success can be judged only by measurements of your body's response to treatment as, unfortunately, if you have diabetes, the fact that you feel well does not mean that you are well controlled. It is only when control goes badly wrong that you may be aware that something is amiss. If your blood glucose is too low, you may be aware of hypo symptoms – if left untreated this may progress to unconsciousness (hypoglycaemic coma). At the other end of the spectrum, when the blood glucose concentration rises very steeply, you may be aware of increased thirst and urination – left untreated, this may progress to nausea, vomiting, weakness, and eventual clouding of consciousness and coma. It has long been apparent that relying on how you feel is too imprecise, even though some people may be able to 'feel' subtle changes in their control. For this reason, many different tests have been developed to allow precise measurement of control and, as the years go by, these tests get better and better.

The involvement of the person with diabetes in monitoring and control of their own condition has always been essential for successful treatment. With the development of blood glucose monitoring, this has become even more apparent: it allows you to measure precisely how effective you are at balancing the conflicting forces of diet, exercise and insulin, and to make adjustments in order to maintain this balance. In the early days after the discovery of insulin, urine tests were the only tests available and it required a small laboratory even to do these. Urine tests have always had the disadvantage in that they are only an indirect indicator of what you really need to know, which is the level of glucose in the blood. Blood glucose monitoring first became available to people with diabetes in 1977 and since then has become widely accepted. As anyone who has monitored glucose levels in the blood will know, these vary considerably throughout the day as well as from day to day. For this reason, a single reading at a twice yearly visit to the local diabetes clinic is of limited value in assessing long-term success or failure with control.

The introduction of haemoglobin A_{1c} (glycosylated haemoglobin or HbA_{1c}) and fructosamine measurements has given a very reliable test for longer term monitoring of average blood glucose levels (taking into account the peaks and troughs) over an interval of 2 to 3 weeks in the case of fructosamine, and of 2 to 3 months for HbA_{1c}. Attaining a normal HbA_{1c} level indicates that the blood glucose concentration has been contained within the normal range, and also that (provided that there are no unacceptable attacks of hypoglycaemia) balance is excellent and no further changes are required. It can be seen that attaining a normal HbA_{1c} level and maintaining it as near normal as possible is an important goal. Not everyone can achieve this, but it is undoubtedly the most effective way of eliminating the risk of long-term complications, as has been proven for Type 1 diabetes in the Diabetes Control and Complications Trial (DCCT) in the USA. In this painstaking study over 1400 people with Type 1 diabetes were divided into two groups, depending on how closely they controlled their blood glucose, and then followed up for an average of 7 years.

The group with good control, with an average HbA_{1c} of 7.2% (see the section on *Haemoglobin A_{1c}* later in this chapter for an explanation of this measurement) benefited from a 60% reduction in disease of the eyes, kidneys and nerves compared with the group with worse control. To achieve this degree of control, the people in this group had four daily injections or received insulin via a constant infusion pump. They also had considerable support from a team of diabetes specialists, including nurse educators, dietitians, psychologists and doctors.

Why monitor?

I developed diabetes at the age of 56 and am struggling to control my sugars with tablets. However, I feel perfectly well and wonder why my doctor is so keen for me to have good control.

In the introduction to this section, we described the DCCT – a large American study, which proved the importance of good control in Type 1 diabetes. Until 1998, there was some doubt about the need for tight control of blood glucose in Type 2 diabetes, which is the most common sort of diabetes developing later in life. The results of a large British research project – the UK Prospective Diabetes Study (UKPDS) – were then published, and provided that clear evidence that the risk of complications in Type 2 diabetes was higher in those people with higher levels of blood glucose and thus of HbA_{1c}. The 5000 people with diabetes in the study were randomly divided into two groups, one with tight control and the other with higher blood sugars. The group with tighter control had 25% less eye disease and 16% less risk of a heart attack.

The UKPDS also proved that, in people with Type 2 diabetes, it is important to keep very strict control of blood pressure. The study also showed that, in most cases, Type 2 diabetes gets steadily worse year on year, which explains why many people end up needing insulin after a few years, even though they are well controlled on tablets at the beginning.

Monitoring other aspects of health is also an important part of long-term diabetes care. Regular checks on eyes, blood pressure, feet and cholesterol are a good way of picking up conditions that require treatment at a stage before they have done any serious damage (long-term complications are covered in Chapter 9). The control of your diabetes is important as is the detection and treatment of any complications, so make sure you are getting the medical care and education that you need to stay healthy. Diabetes UK have published a guide called *What diabetes care to expect*, which we have reprinted in the section on **Diabetes clinics** later in this chapter.

I am an 18-year-old on insulin. When my glucose is high I do not feel any ill effects. Is it really necessary for me to maintain strict control?

It is quite true that some people do not develop the typical thirst or dry mouth, frequency of passing water (urination), or tiredness, which usually occur if the blood glucose is high and diabetes out of control. It sounds as if you are one of these people, which makes it much more difficult for you to sense when your control is poor and take steps to improve it. Yet even without these symptoms, control of your blood glucose is still important. The development of complications after many years is much less likely (and may possibly be eliminated) if you can maintain blood glucose concentrations within the normal range. We know that it is difficult at 18 to be concerned about things that might only happen a long time ahead in your future, but good control really is worth it in the long run.

My 17-year-old daughter has had diabetes for 6 years. She is finding it very difficult to keep her diabetes under control at present and doesn't seem to care if her sugars run high most of the time. Do you think she is doing herself any real damage?

There is now hard proof that good control of blood glucose reduces the risk of developing the complications of diabetes (which are dealt with in Chapter 9). In September 1993 the findings of the Diabetes Control and Complications Trial (known as the DCCT) were published and showed that good control did reduce complications (see the introduction to this chapter). This improvement in control was accompanied by a 3-fold increase in the risk of hypos, and occasionally these hypos required help from someone else to bring the person round.

Thus your daughter is faced with a difficult decision. If she carries on with poor control, she increases her chance of developing long-term problems from her diabetes. If, on the other hand, she decides to try and improve her blood glucose levels, she may have more hypos. In practice, it is worth spending time with your daughter discussing the problem with sensitivity rather than facing her with a stark choice. She needs to be given time to make up her own mind, but remember that occasional hypos do not do any lasting harm so long as they are not frequent or severe. Most people with good control of their diabetes accept that they may have hypos.

Whenever I go to the clinic I always feel guilty for not doing enough blood tests. In fact I sometimes feel like writing in some make-believe tests into my testing book just to keep the doctors happy.

Writing make-believe tests in your book won't keep your doctors happy and, more importantly, won't help you stop feeling guilty about not doing your blood tests. What might help is looking at some possible reasons why you are not doing the tests.

When you first went on insulin you were probably the centre of attention with support from your family, school friends or workmates. You probably had close contact with a diabetes specialist nurse to help you through a difficult time. During this period, measuring your blood glucose became a routine occurrence so that you could adjust your dose of insulin. After a few months, this phase of intense attention passed and you may have decided on a fixed insulin dose, only to be varied in unusual circumstances.

It can be depressing when the initial interest fades and you have to come to terms with the fact that the routine of diabetes is for keeps. This is a time when people may give up testing their blood glucose except when they feel ill. We have interviewed a number of people who have given up testing and the most common reasons they gave for giving up are as follows:

- Testing is messy and bloody.
- I haven't got time/can't be bothered to test my blood.
- There is no need to test if you feel all right.
- Testing my blood brings it home to me that I have diabetes.
- It is inconvenient/embarrassing testing in public or at work.
- Insulin injections are essential, blood tests are not.
- A bad test makes me feel even more depressed about my diabetes.
- There is no point in testing my blood as I don't use the information.

These are the opinions of people living with diabetes and they must be respected. You might like to think where you stand on this subject, and perhaps discuss it with someone on your next clinic visit. We feel that, if you need insulin, you will only achieve good control by doing regular blood tests since there is no other way of knowing how you are doing.

In the past 12 months I have had to increase my insulin dosage several times, yet I was still unable to get a blood test result that was near normal. I have had diabetes for 25 years and until last year I have always been well controlled. What has gone wrong?

Here are a few reasons why your blood glucose levels may have crept up and why you need more insulin after many years of good control:

- less exercise, meaning that more insulin is needed for your food intake;
- an increase in your diet;
- increased stress or emotional upsets;
- any illness that tends to linger on, leading to a need for more insulin;
- technical problems with injections such as the appearance of lumps from repeated doses of insulin into the same site;
- increase in weight and middle-age spread.

Having said all that, some people do find that the dose of insulin that they need may vary by quite large amounts for no obvious reason.

Can stress influence blood glucose readings?

Yes, but the response varies from one person to another. In some people stress tends to make the blood glucose rise whereas in other people it may increase the risk of hypoglycaemia.

Would I be able to achieve better control if I went onto three injections a day?

Probably. Most people on multiple injections use an insulin pen, which is more convenient than a syringe. In some cases this has improved control, but studies carried out so far show that not all people have necessarily shown an improvement. However, people like the basal + bolus (multiple injection) regimen because it makes mealtimes more flexible and frees them from having to eat at fixed times. There is a section on *Insulin pens* in Chapter 3.

Blood glucose testing

What is the normal range of blood glucose in a person who does not have diabetes?

Before meals the range is from 3.5 to 5.5 mmol/litre. After meals it may rise as high as 10 mmol/litre depending on the carbohydrate content of the meal. However long a person without diabetes goes without food, the blood glucose concentration never drops below 3 mmol/litre, and however much they eat, it never goes above 10 mmol/litre.

My blood glucose monitor is calculated in millimoles. Can you tell me what a millimole is?

In the 1960s, international agreement led to scientists in most parts of the world using a standard system of metric measurements. The units are called SI units, an abbreviation of their full name – the 'Système International d'Unites'. There are several units, many of which you probably use without thinking about them, such as the metre. The unit for an amount of a substance is called a mole; the prefix milli- means one thousandth, so a millimole is one thousandth of a mole. Blood glucose is measured in millimoles of glucose per litre of blood, and this is abbreviated to mmol/litre.

Before SI units were introduced, blood glucose was measured in milligrams per 100 millilitres of blood (abbreviated to mg% or to mg per dl) and this measurement is still used in the USA. The table below shows how one set of units relates to the other.

1 mmol/litre = 18 mg%	9 mmol/litre = 162 mg%
2 mmol/litre = 36 mg%	10 mmol/litre = 180 mg%
3 mmol/litre = 54 mg%	12 mmol/litre = 216 mg%
4 mmol/litre = 72 mg%	15 mmol/litre = 270 mg%
5 mmol/litre = 90 mg%	20 mmol/litre = 360 mg%
6 mmol/litre = 108 mg%	22 mmol/litre = 396 mg%
7 mmol/litre = 126 mg%	25 mmol/litre = 450 mg%
8 mmol/litre = 144 mg%	30 mmol/litre = 540 mg%

Is blood glucose monitoring suitable for people whose diabetes is controlled by tablets?

Yes, it is. Everyone with diabetes, whether controlled by diet, diet and tablets, or insulin, should strive for perfect control. Traditionally this has been achieved by regular urine tests at home. Since 1977 there has been a move towards encouraging people to do their own blood glucose measurements. This form of monitoring was first thought to be most suitable for insulin-treated people. However, further experience has shown that it is equally suited to those treated with diet and tablets. The disadvantage of having to prick your finger to obtain a drop of blood is more than compensated for by the increased accuracy and reliability of the readings so obtained.

Should I keep my sticks for blood glucose monitoring in the fridge with my insulin?

No. It is important to keep them dry as any moisture will impair their activity. You must put the lid back on the container immediately after removing a strip (unless the strips are individually foil-wrapped). Many of the strips contain enzymes, which are biological substances that do not last forever, and the sticks should never be used beyond their expiry date. The bottle of sticks should be kept in a cool, dry place, and should not be exposed to extremely high temperatures. If you have any reason to suspect the result of a blood test, the best thing is to repeat the test using a new bottle of strips.

I had a glucose tolerance test and my highest blood glucose was 17 mmol/litre. However, my urine analysis was negative for glucose. Is there a way I could test my blood for glucose without going to the laboratory?

You appear to have a 'high renal threshold' to glucose (see the section on *Urine testing* later in this chapter for more information about this), which means that it is only at very high concentrations of glucose in the blood that any glucose escapes into your urine. In your case urine tests are unhelpful and blood tests essential. Nowadays most people monitor their blood glucose using the compact and convenient meters that are widely available.

There are several different blood testing techniques. Although a few can be read by eye, it is possible to make this reading more effective by use of a specially designed meter. Most strips can be used only with a specific meter.

Most hospital diabetes clinics will be able to show you the various strips and meters that are available, and your choice should be made after discussion with your diabetes specialist nurse or doctor in the clinic. All the different methods give good results provided that they are used sensibly and after proper instruction. The blood glucose meters are not available on prescription, but the strips are.

There is more information about both strips and meters later in this section, and a list of meters currently available is in Appendix 1.

I feel hypo when my blood glucose is normal and only well when it is high. I feel very ill when my doctor tries to keep my blood glucose normal. Am I hooked on a high blood glucose?

In someone who has had poor control for several years, the brain and other tissues in the body can adjust themselves to a high concentration of glucose in the blood. As a result they may feel hypo at a time when their blood glucose is normal or even high. The long-term outlook for such people is not good unless they can re-educate themselves to tolerate normal blood glucose levels without feeling unwell. This is possible but requires determination and an understanding of the long-term dangers of a high blood glucose.

Your problem can be overcome by regular measurement of blood glucose, but you must accept that, however unwell you feel, no harm will be done if your blood glucose remains above 4 mmol/litre. It may take up to 6 months of good control for this feeling to wear off, but it will be worth it.

Is there a way of knowing how much extra Actrapid insulin to give depending on my blood glucose level so I can maintain a better blood glucose?

The answer is yes, but it will require some experimenting on your part. The particular type and dose of insulin most suited to you can best be judged by repeated measurements of your body's response to the insulin you are taking. If you find, for example, that your blood glucose always goes very high after breakfast, then you may be able to prevent this by taking more Actrapid before breakfast but, before making any adjustment in insulin dosage, it is important to see that the blood glucose changes that you see are part of a regular pattern. This is part of the process of balancing insulin, diet and exercise, and we would caution against taking an extra dose of insulin if you come across a rather high blood glucose reading as an isolated finding. It is usually far better to try to work out a routine whereby you can prevent your blood glucose from rising too high rather than to take an extra injection of insulin after it has happened. There are exceptions to this rule, of course. If you suddenly become unwell and your blood glucose goes very high, repeated extra injections of a short-acting insulin such as Actrapid or Novorapid are the most effective way of preventing the development of keto-acidosis (see the *Glossary* for an explanation of this serious condition).

Are there any general guidelines for insulin adjustment?

This will really depend on the type of insulin you are taking, and the number of injections you have each day. We give three examples in Table 4.1.

The general rule is to increase your insulin by 2 units at a time and to leave the dose as it is for a few days to see if the results improve. The exception to this is at times of illness and infection, when the dose may need to be increased by 4–10 units, sometimes with additional doses of short-acting insulin given between the usual injection times until the blood glucose levels start to improve.

The dose of insulin will need to be reduced if hypos occur regularly.

I find that my control is only good for 1 week a month and that is the week before my period. Why is this and what should I do about it?

In some women the dose of insulin required to control diabetes varies in relation to the menstrual cycle. Your question implies that you become more sensitive to insulin in the week before you menstruate and you probably require more insulin at the other times in your cycle. There is no reason why you should not try to work out a pattern where you reduce your insulin dose in the week before your period and increase it at other times.

The variation is due to different hormones coming from the ovaries during the menstrual cycle. Some of these hormones have an anti-insulin effect. The same sort of effects may occur when a woman is taking oral contraceptive tablets (the pill) or is pregnant. The correct thing to do is to make adjustments in the insulin dose in order to compensate for these hormonal changes and to keep the balance of the blood glucose where it should be.

I have noticed that there are much greater fluctuations in my blood glucose level when I am having a period. I have great difficulty in keeping my blood glucose balanced then. I have read many books on diabetes but I have never seen this mentioned – is it normal?

It is quite normal for the blood glucose control to fluctuate during the monthly cycle. Most women find their blood glucose is highest in the premenstrual phase and returns to normal during or after their period. Some women need to adjust their dose of insulin during the cycle but rarely by more than a few units. Every woman has to discover for herself the extent of this effect and how much extra insulin, if any, is needed. Your diabetes clinic doctor or diabetes specialist nurse is the best person to turn to for exact advice on how to make these adjustments.

Table 4.1 Insulin adjustment

Intermediate-acting insulin (e.g. Humulin I, Insulatard, Monotard) taken twice a day

IF YOUR BLOOD GLUCOSE IS TOO HIGH			
BEFORE BREAKFAST	BEFORE LUNCH	BEFORE DINNER	BEFORE BED
Increase p.m. insulin	Increase a.m. insulin	Increase a.m. insulin	Increase p.m. insulin

Short-acting insulin (e.g. Actrapid, Velosulin, Humulin S) taken with intermediate-acting insulin twice a day

IF YOUR BLOOD GLUCOSE IS TOO HIGH			
BEFORE BREAKFAST	BEFORE LUNCH	BEFORE DINNER	BEFORE BED
Increase p.m. intermediate insulin	Increase a.m. short insulin	Increase a.m. intermediate insulin	Increase p.m. short insulin

Short-acting insulin taken three times a day, before meals, with intermediate- or long-acting insulin at bedtime

IF YOUR BLOOD GLUCOSE IS TOO HIGH			
BEFORE BREAKFAST	BEFORE LUNCH	BEFORE DINNER	BEFORE BED
Increase bedtime insulin	Increase breakfast short insulin	Increase lunchtime short insulin	Increase dinnertime short insulin

Where is the best place to obtain blood for measuring blood glucose levels?

It is usually easiest to obtain blood from the fingertips. You can use either the pulp, which is the fleshy part of the fingertip, or the sides of the fingertips. Some people like to use the area just below the nail bed. Most people find it easier to use the tip but the sides of the fingertips are less sensitive than the pulp. It may be necessary for some people such as guitarists, pianists or typists to avoid the finger pulp.

The fleshy ear lobes are also suitable areas for obtaining blood and are less sensitive than the fingers but they can be difficult to use as the blood has to be applied to the reagent stick with the use of a mirror. Parents may find that it is easiest to obtain blood from the earlobes of their child with diabetes. There are a couple of meters that allow blood to be taken from the arm. (See a later question in this chapter).

Which is the best finger pricker?

All the currently available blood lancets are very similar and there is very little to choose between any of them. The lancets may be used either on their own or in conjunction with an automatic device. They are obtainable on prescription from your own GP. Alternatively they can be bought from a chemist, or sent for by post from companies such as Owen Mumford (Medical Shop) – see Appendix 3 for addresses.

If you have trouble pricking your fingers without an automatic finger pricker, there are now a wealth of devices that make the task much easier. These are all very similar and work on the principle of hiding the lancet from view whilst piercing the skin very quickly and at a controlled depth. They are not available on prescription, but can be purchased from chemists, or by post from companies such as Owen Mumford (Medical Shop). There are too many devices to list here, but the latest products are advertised in *Balance*, the magazine published by Diabetes UK.

Before buying any automatic finger pricker, check that you are using the correct lancets with the appropriate finger pricker, as some are not interchangeable. Your health professional will be able to advise you. Some manufacturers offer finger prickers as part of the package when you buy a meter.

Should I clean my fingers with spirit or antiseptic before pricking them?

We do not recommend the use of spirit for cleaning your fingers as its constant use will lead to hardening of the skin of your fingertips. It can also interfere with the reagent strips. We suggest that you wash your hands with soap and warm water and dry them thoroughly before pricking your finger.

Will constant finger pricking make my fingers sore?

You may find that your fingers feel sore for the first week or two after starting blood glucose monitoring but this soon disappears. We have seen many people who have been measuring their blood glucose levels regularly 3 or 4 times a day for more than 15 years and who have no problems with sore fingers. Don't always use the same finger – instead try to use different fingers in rotation.

Will my fingers take a long time to heal after finger pricking and am I more likely to pick up an infection there?

Your fingertips should heal as quickly as someone without diabetes but make sure that you are using suitable blood lancets. We have seen only one infected finger among many hundreds of thousands of finger pricks. We suggest that you keep your hands socially clean and wash them before collecting your blood sample.

There are a bewildering number of blood glucose sticks and meters on the market. Which are the best to use?

This is purely a matter of preference and may depend on the type of strips or meters used in your local clinic.

Some strips require wiping or blotting and are then compared with a colour chart after careful timing, whilst others do not need wiping or blotting, and can only be used with a meter. There is a list of currently available meters in Appendix 1. The magazine *Balance*, produced by Diabetes UK, usually carries advertisements for the latest strips and meters, and their use should be discussed with your diabetes specialist nurse or diabetes physician. Blood glucose testing strips are obtainable on prescription from your GP but the meters have to be purchased, although many are now quite inexpensive.

I have recently started using BM-Test strips but have been told that my results do not compare well with the hospital results. What is the reason for this?

The first thing to do is to make sure that your technique is absolutely correct. Inaccurate results will be obtained if the correct procedures are not followed completely. If your technique is not at fault, then it could be that you are not able to interpret the colour chart correctly. If this is so, you would be advised to use a meter, which reads the blood glucose result for you.

My blood glucose meter appears to give slightly different results compared with the hospital laboratory. Are the meters accurate enough for daily use?

Most results obtained when you are using a meter will be slightly different from the hospital laboratory results because different chemical methods are used. These slight differences do not matter and the strips and meters are quite accurate enough for home use.

If your results are very different from the laboratory, it could be that your technique is incorrect. The most common fault is not applying a large enough drop of blood to the strip. Other faults are smearing the blood on the strip, or taking too long to apply the blood to the strip. The reaction must also be timed accurately. The insert or carrier of the meter must be kept clean, and you should follow the maker's instructions for cleaning the carrier. Also check that the reagent strips are not used past their expiry date. If all else fails, read the instructions!

I have trouble obtaining enough blood to cover the whole test pad on the strip. Is there anything that I can do to make this easier?

If you are having trouble obtaining enough blood, you might find the use of an automatic finger pricker makes it easier. Also try to warm your hands by washing them in warm water before you start, and drying them thoroughly before pricking your finger. Finally, when squeezing the blood out of your finger, try 'milking' the blood out gently, allowing the finger to recover in between each squeeze. Do not squeeze so hard that you end up 'blanching' the finger. Many of the strips that are used with modern meters require very little blood, and your diabetes team should be able to advise you on these.

I understand that there is a combined blood glucose meter and lancet. Can you tell me more about it?

You are probably referring to the Soft-Sense from MediSense. This is a blood glucose meter that has the facility for also pricking the skin. A lancet is inserted into the meter, the meter is placed on the arm, the skin is pricked, and a vacuum draws up the blood onto the sample area of the test strip. After 20 seconds the vacuum is released, the Soft-Sense is removed from the skin, and the result is then shown on the screen and stored in the meter's memory. One of its advantages is that different areas of the arm can be used for testing, but it has the disadvantage of being expensive.

I am about to buy a meter that allows blood to be taken from the arm. Are there any problems with arm testing?

At the time of writing there are three meters that allow blood testing to be taken from the arm. One is the Soft-Sense (see question above), the others are the OneTouch Ultra from LifeScan and the FreeStyle from TheraSense. The OneTouch Ultra and FreeStyle use strips that allow a tiny blood sample to be taken, which makes arm testing feasible. Under certain conditions, samples taken from the arm may differ significantly from fingertip samples, such as when blood glucose is changing rapidly following a meal, after an insulin dose or when taking physical exercise. Arm samples should only be used for testing prior to, or more than 2 hours after meals, insulin dose or physical exercise. Fingertip testing should be used whenever there is a concern about hypoglycaemia (such as when you drive a car), as arm testing may fail to detect an insulin reaction. The elderly can have problems obtaining sufficient blood from the arm. Your health professional should be consulted before you begin arm testing.

I have heard that there is a way of obtaining blood from a finger using a laser. Is this true?

The Lasette is a single shot laser that makes a small hole in the finger to obtain a drop of blood, but it is not a blood glucose monitoring device. The use of laser light, as opposed to a steel lancet, reduces tissue damage, and many users of the device report feeling less pain than when using a traditional lancet. It weighs just less than 260 g (9 oz). However, it is very expensive. It is slightly smaller than a videocassette. The Lasette is manufactured by Cell Robotics, and can be obtained from Nutech International, whose address is listed in Appendix 3.

I would like to measure my own blood glucose levels, but as I am now blind I do not know if this is possible. Can it be done?

Unfortunately, this is no longer possible as manufacturers have stopped making 'talking' meters. Maybe you could get a friend to help you.

Urine

**I do not understand why it is that the glucose from the
blood only spills into the urine above a certain level. I
gather this level is known as the renal threshold – could
you explain it for me in a little more detail?**

Urine is formed by filtration of blood in the kidneys. When the
glucose concentration in the blood is below about 10 mmol/litre,
any glucose filtered into the urine is subsequently reabsorbed
back into the bloodstream. When the level of glucose exceeds
about 10 mmol/litre (the renal threshold) more glucose is filtered
than the body can reabsorb, and as a result it is passed in the
urine. Once the level has exceeded 10 mmol/litre, the amount of
glucose in the urine will be proportional to the level of glucose in
the blood. Below 10 mmol/litre, however, there will be no glucose
in the urine and, since the blood glucose level never exceeds 10
mmol/litre in people without diabetes, they will not find glucose
in the urine, unless they have a particular inherited condition
called renal glycosuria.

**How do you know if you have ketones in your urine? What
are they and are they dangerous?**

Ketones are breakdown products of the fat stores in the body.
They are present in small amounts even in people without diabetes, particularly when they are dieting or fasting and therefore
relying on their body fat stores for energy. In people with diabetes
small amounts of ketones in the urine are commonly found. They
become dangerous only when they are present in large amounts.
This is usually accompanied by thirst, passing large amounts of
urine, and nausea. If ketones are present in the urine together
with continuous 2% glucose, or blood glucose levels higher than
13 mmol/litre, then they are dangerous as this is the condition that
precedes the development of ketoacidosis. **Under these circumstances you should seek urgent medical advice.**
    You can test your urine for ketones with strips such as

Ketur-Test or Keto Diabur; the latter tests for glucose as well and both are made by Roche; or Ketostix or KetoDiastix (made by Bayer Diagnostics) – they are all available on prescription from your GP. MediSense produce an Optium meter that tests for blood glucose and blood ketones but, although the glucose testing strips are available on prescription, the blood ketone strips are not.

What does it mean if I have a lot of ketones but no glucose on urine testing?

Testing for ketones in the urine can be rather confusing and, unless there are special reasons for doing it, we do not recommend it for routine use. Some people seem to develop ketones in the urine very readily, especially children, pregnant women and people who are dieting strictly to lose weight.

Usually if glucose and ketones appear together it indicates poor diabetes control, although this may be transient, and glucose and ketones, present in the morning, may disappear by noon. If they persist all the time, then control almost certainly needs to be improved, probably by increasing the insulin dose.

Ketones do sometimes appear in the urine without glucose, although not very frequently. They are most commonly seen in the first morning specimen and probably occur as the insulin action from the night before is wearing off – in some people the ketone levels increase before the glucose levels. Under these circumstances it is not serious and no particular action is needed.

Finally, ketones without glucose in the urine are very common in people who are trying to lose weight through calorie restriction. Anyone who is on a strict diet and losing weight will burn up body fat and this causes ketones to appear in the urine. Provided that there is no excess glucose in your urine, these ketones do not mean that your diabetes is out of control.

Why do we not always get a true blood glucose reading through a urine test (as in my case)?

In most people urine contains glucose only when the glucose concentration in the blood is higher than a certain figure (usually

10 mmol/litre), so below this level urine tests give no indication at all of the concentration of glucose in the blood. The level at which glucose spills out into the urine (the renal threshold – discussed earlier in this section) varies from one person to another and you can assess it in yourself only by making many simultaneous blood and urine glucose measurements. If you undertake this exercise you will undoubtedly find, like most other people, that the relationship between the blood and urine concentrations is not very precise. For this reason most people nowadays prefer to do blood tests rather than urine tests, as they find that the increased precision of blood tests outweighs any disadvantage that may stem from having to prick your finger to get a drop of blood.

For some time now I have suffered from diabetes. I am always curious to know what type of tests are made on my urine specimens when they are taken off to the laboratory.

Urine specimens are tested for several things but the most common are glucose, ketones and albumin (protein). These tests serve only as a spot check and are meant to complement your own tests performed at home. Clinics like to know the percentage of glucose in samples taken at different times of day as giving some measure of control at home. The detection of ketones is of rather limited value since some people make ketones very easily and others almost not at all, but the presence of large amounts of ketones together with 2% glucose shows that the person is very badly out of control. The presence of protein in the urine can indicate either infection in the urine or the presence of some kidney disease, which in people with diabetes is likely to be diabetic nephropathy, one of the long-term complications (see Chapter 9 for more information about this). A more recent test is for microalbuminuria – the test detects microscopic amounts of albumin in the urine and can show signs of very early kidney damage.

I have a strong family history of diabetes. My daughter recently tested her urine and found 2% glucose. However, her blood glucose was only 8 mmol/litre. She underwent a glucose tolerance test and this was normal. Could she have diabetes or could there be another reason why she is passing glucose in her water?

It is very unlikely that she has diabetes if a glucose tolerance test was normal. If she had glucose in her urine during the glucose tolerance test when all the blood glucose readings were strictly normal, then this would indicate that she has a low renal threshold for glucose (as discussed at the beginning of this section). If this is the correct diagnosis, then it is important to find out whether she passes glucose in her urine first thing in the morning while fasting or only after she has eaten. In people who pass glucose in their urine during the fasting state, there is not known to be any increased incidence of development of diabetes, and the condition (called renal glycosuria) is inherited. If, on the other hand, she passes glucose in the urine only after meals containing starch and sugar, this condition sometimes progresses to diabetes.

Haemoglobin A_{1c} and fructosamine

When I last went to the clinic, I had a test for haemoglobin A_{1c}. What is this for and what are the normal values?

Haemoglobin A_{1c} is a component of the red pigment (haemoglobin A; HbA) present in the blood to carry oxygen from the lungs to the various organs in the body. The HbA_{1c} can be measured as a percentage of all the haemoglobin present with a variety of laboratory methods. HbA_{1c} consists of HbA combined with glucose by a chemical link. The amount of HbA_{1c} present is directly proportional to the average blood glucose during the 120-day lifespan of the HbA-containing red blood corpuscles in the circulating blood.

It is the most successful of all the tests so far developed to give an index of diabetes control. The blood glucose tests, which we have used for many years, fluctuate too erratically with injections, meals and other events for an isolated sample taken at one clinic visit to provide much information about overall control. HbA_{1c} averages out the peaks and troughs of the blood glucose over the previous 2 to 3 months.

Normal values vary a little from one laboratory to another and this can be a source of confusion as results from different clinics cannot be compared directly without the normal range known for each particular laboratory. (Diabetes UK is trying to correct this anomaly.) Normal values usually run between 4.5% and 6.1%, but you must check the normal range for your own laboratory. In someone with poorly controlled diabetes, or in whom diabetes is recently diagnosed, the value of HbA_{1c} may be as high as 15%, which reflects a consistently raised blood glucose over the preceding 2 to 3 months. On the other hand, in someone with perfect control, the HbA_{1c} will be in the normal range of 4.5–6.1%, while in someone who runs blood glucose levels too low owing to taking too much insulin, the value will be subnormal, i.e. below 6%. Recently HbA_{1c} has replaced HbA_1 as the preferred terminology. It refers to a subcomponent of HbA_1, which most closely represents the indicator of average blood glucose level over two months.

I've just had a fructosamine test but I didn't like to ask what this was for. What is this test?

Fructosamine is the name of a test that is similar to that for HbA_{1c} in that it is an indicator of the average level of glucose in the blood over a period of time, in this case the 2 to 3 weeks before the test is done (compared with the preceding 2 to 3 months for HbA_{1c}). It measures the amount of glucose linked to the proteins in the blood plasma (the straw-coloured fluid in which the red cells are suspended): the higher the blood glucose concentration, the higher will be the fructosamine. Its advantages are that it is usually quicker and cheaper for the laboratory to do. The normal values may vary from one laboratory to another depending on the way the analysis is performed; in general, a value of less than 300 micromol/litre is a typical laboratory's normal value. In order to make sure you don't get confused, we suggest that you pay particular attention to what is done in your clinic; please don't hesitate to ask and make quite sure you do know what is going on!

Will this test have to be done regularly?

Like HbA_{1c} there is no point in doing them too often; we normally recommend doing one routinely at the time of each clinic visit. If metabolic control is under close scrutiny and treatment is being adjusted, for example in pregnancy, then it may be sensible to do one more often to check that things are going according to plan.

I am 25 years old and have had diabetes since I was 15. I have been attending the clinic regularly every 3 months and do regular blood glucose tests at home with my own meter. At my last clinic visit, the doctor I saw said that he did not need to see me again for a whole year because my HbA_{1c} was consistently normal – why did he do this?

It sounds as though your specialist has great confidence in you and your ability to control your diabetes. As long as you can keep it this way, he clearly feels that seeing you once a year is sufficient. He can then spend more time with other people who are not as successful as you are.

I am treated only by diet. I find it very difficult to stick to my diet or do the tests between the clinic visits but I am always very strict for the few days before I am seen at the clinic and my blood glucose test is usually normal. At my last clinic visit my blood glucose was 5 mmol/litre but the doctor said he was very unhappy about my control because the HbA_{1c} was too high at 10% – what did he mean?

Your experience demonstrates the usefulness of HbA_{1c} testing, because you have been misleading yourself as well as your medical advisers about your ability to cope with your diabetes. The HbA$_{1c}$ has brought this to the surface for the first time. Because the HbA$_{1c}$ reflects what your blood glucose has been doing for as long as 2 to 3 months before your clinic visit, your last minute attempts to get your diabetes under control before you went to the clinic were enough to bring the blood glucose down but the HbA$_{1c}$ remained high.

My recent HbA$_{1c}$ was said to be low at 6%. Blood glucose readings look all right, on average about 5 mmol/litre. The specialist asked me to set the alarm clock and check them at 3.00am – why is this?

A low HbA$_{1c}$ suggests that at some stage your blood glucose levels are running unduly low. If you are not having hypo-glycaemic attacks during the day, then it is possible that they are occurring at night and you are sleeping through them. By doing 3.00am blood glucose tests you should be able to determine whether this is so. Incidentally, you will only have to do these middle-of-the-night tests until you have established whether or not you are having hypos at night – they are not going to be a per-manent part of your routine!

My diabetes is treated with diet and gliclazide tablets. By strict dieting I have lost weight down to slightly below my target figure and all my urine tests are negative. My HbA$_{1c}$ test, I am told, is still too high at 9% and does not seem to be falling despite the fact that I am still losing weight. I could not tolerate metformin and am very strict over what I eat. At the last clinic visit the doctor said that I am going to have to go on to insulin injections. I have been dreading these all my life – is he right?

The high HbA$_{1c}$ means that your average blood glucose result is not well controlled and it sounds very much as if you have reached the stage where you need more than gliclazide and diet to keep your diabetes under good control. You could try an addi-tional tablet such as rosiglitazone but, if this fails, you will need to move on to the next stronger form of treatment, which is insulin injections. You have been given sound advice and we are sure that it will not turn out to be as bad as you imagine. Once you have got over the initial fear of injecting yourself, which most people manage very quickly, you will probably feel a great deal better and it will all have been worthwhile.

Diabetes clinics

They have just appointed a new young consultant at my hospital and I am told that they are going to start a special diabetes clinic – will this offer any advantage to me?

Most hospitals these days have at least one senior doctor who specializes in diabetes. By running a special diabetes clinic they can bring together all the specially trained doctors, nurses, dietitians and chiropodists, and this should mean a better service for you and other people attending the clinic. You will have the benefit of seeing people who have special training in diabetes, and most people find this a big advantage.

My GP is starting a diabetes clinic in the local group practice and tells me that I no longer need to attend the hospital clinic. It's much more convenient for me to go to see my GP but will this be all right?

You are fortunate that your general practitioner has a special interest in diabetes and has gone to the trouble of setting up a special clinic in the practice for this. Many GPs and practice nurses have had special training in diabetes and these general practice-based diabetes clinics are becoming more common. We are sure that your hospital specialist will know about this, and may even attend the GP clinic from time to time. If you have any anxieties, why not discuss it with your doctor? Many GPs now like to look after people with diabetes in general practice without the need to visit hospital. This is usually all right as long as you have uncomplicated diabetes and are well controlled, but you should be aware of the sort of care that you should expect – we have reprinted Diabetes UK's recommendations on this at the end of this section.

Although they do a blood test every time I go to our local diabetes clinic, they now only test my urine once a year when they look at my eyes and check my blood pressure – why is this?

With the introduction of HbA_{1c} measurement and blood glucose monitoring, the value of urine testing is really for the detection of protein (albumin) in the urine as an indicator of possible kidney damage. This does not need to be done more often than once a year in people who are quite well and free from albumin in their urine. As a general rule everyone with diabetes should have their urine, eyes, feet and blood pressure checked annually.

Why do I have to wait such a long time every time I go to the diabetes clinic?

If you think about it, you probably have quite a lot of tests done when you go to the clinic. It takes time to get the answers back and the results all together before you see the doctor. This is particularly likely to be so if you have had a blood glucose measurement, as the HbA_{1c} levels measured in the clinic take time to process. Although it may be irritating to have to wait for these results, they are very important as they can be used in a two-way discussion between you and the doctor to review your control and progress with diabetes. Many clinics use this waiting time for showing educational films or videos about diabetes and for meeting the dietitian and/or chiropodist, as well as the diabetes specialist nurse. If the clinic appears to be badly organized then you have good grounds for complaint.

What determines whether my next appointment is in 1 month or 6 months?

Generally speaking, if your control is consistently good you will not need to be seen very often; on the other hand, if your control is poor it is likely that you will be seen more often. This is not, as you may perhaps think, a subtle form of punishment, but it will give you and your medical advisers more opportunity to sort out what is wrong.

At my clinic we have a mixture of people from young children to very old pensioners – why do they not have special clinics for young people?

Young people with diabetes have special needs, which are not usually met by an ordinary diabetes clinic. Growing up and learning to be independent places extra strains on diabetes control and young people prefer a more informal approach from members of the diabetes team. Some hospitals find it difficult to make these changes and there may be extra costs. However, clinics for young people have been set up in many parts of the country and you could ask your GP if you could be referred to one of them.

We have a specialist nurse in diabetes working in the diabetes clinic that I attend. What does she do?

Most clinics in this country now employ specialist nurses who spend their whole time working with people with diabetes. They may work in the community and/or the hospital and have a variety of titles – Diabetic Health Visitor, Diabetic Community Nurse, Diabetic or Diabetes Liaison Nurse, Diabetes Specialist Nurse, Diabetes Sister, Diabetic or Diabetes Care Sister, etc. These senior nurses spend most of their time educating people, giving advice (much of it on the telephone), making decisions about management and teaching other members of the medical and nursing staff about diabetes. They are experts in their field and are central members of the diabetes care team.

As a newly diagnosed person with diabetes what sort of care should I expect?

Diabetes UK issued a document in June 2000 (from guidelines first produced in 1986) called *What diabetes care to expect*. This document explains clearly what standards of care to expect and as a result we are reprinting the guidelines from it here (see the box overleaf). If you would like a copy of the complete document, contact Diabetes UK (address in Appendix 3).

It seems surprising that the government has not given some clear guidelines about diabetes care.

Yes it is surprising when you consider that over a million people in the UK have diabetes and that it uses up a great deal of NHS money. In fact the Department of Health started to set up such a scheme, called the National Service Framework (NSF) for Diabetes. Similar schemes have already appeared for other branches of medicine such as cardiology and mental health.

Consultations with the NSF for diabetes started in 1999 and the expert committee made its report in April 2001. It was expected that the government would roll out the project by the end of 2001. In October of that year the Minister of Health announced that the plans for diabetes would be released in 2002 but that the programme would take place over 10 years and that funding would start in April 2003. We presume that the NSF for Diabetes has turned out to be much more costly than expected and the government are therefore delaying its launch until they can be sure to fund it.

The first section of the NSF was published in 2001. This consists of the agreed standards and we must wait until April 2003 before the funding for this important project will start to appear. We print the standards in the second box in this chapter; copies of the complete 48 page NSF document can be obtained from Department of Health (see Appendix 3).

We can only hope that the NSF will be adequately funded to cause a real improvement in diabetes care right across the country.

Note also that the National Institute for Clinical Excellence (NICE) has produced detailed guidelines for diabetes care. They deal with blood glucose and (in a separate booklet) blood pressure and lipids. You can get these guidelines off the Internet (www.nice.org.uk) or send for copies to NICE (see Appendix 3).

When you have just been diagnosed you should have:

- a full medical examination;
- a talk with a registered nurse who has a special interest in diabetes; she will explain what diabetes is and talk to you about your individual treatment;
- a talk with a State Registered dietitian, who will want to know what you are used to eating and will give you basic advice on what to eat in future; a follow-up meeting should be arranged for more detailed advice;
- a discussion on the implications of diabetes on your job, driving, insurance, prescription charges, etc.; whether you need to inform the DVLA and your insurance company, if you are a driver;
- information about the Diabetes UK's services and details of your local Diabetes UK group;
- ongoing education about your diabetes and the beneficial effects of exercise, and assessments of your control.

You should be able to take a close friend or relative with you to educational sessions if you wish.

PLUS

If you are treated by insulin, you should receive:

- frequent sessions for basic instruction in injection technique, looking after insulin and syringes or insulin pens, blood glucose and urine ketone testing and what the results mean;
- supplies of relevant equipment;
- discussion about hypoglycaemia (hypos), when and why it may happen and what to do about it.

If you are treated by tablets, you should receive:

- discussion about the possibility of hypoglycaemia (hypos) and how to deal with it;
- instruction on blood or urine testing and what the results mean, and supplies of relevant equipment.

If you are treated by diet alone, you should receive:

- instruction on blood or urine testing and what the results mean, and supplies of relevant equipment.

Once your diabetes is reasonably controlled, you should:

- have access to the diabetes team at regular intervals – annually if necessary; these meetings should give time for discussion as well as assessing diabetes control;
- be able to contact any member of the healthcare team for specialist advice when you need it;
- have more education sessions as you are ready for them;
- have a formal medical review once a year by a doctor experienced in diabetes.

At this review:

- your weight should be recorded;
- your urine should be tested for protein;
- your blood should be tested to measure long-term control;
- you should discuss control, including your home monitoring results and details of any severe hypos;
- your blood pressure should be checked;
- your vision should be checked and the back of your eyes examined with an ophthalmoscope; a photo may be taken of the back of your eyes, and if necessary you should be referred to an ophthalmologist;
- your legs and feet should be examined to check your circulation and nerve supply, and if necessary you should be referred to a State Registered chiropodist;
- if you are on insulin, your injection sites should be examined;
- you should have the opportunity to discuss how you are coping at home and at work.

Your role:

- You are an important member of the care team so it is essential that you understand your own diabetes to enable you to be in control of your condition.
- You should ensure that you receive the described care from your local diabetes clinic, practice or hospital.

If these services are not available to you, you should:

- contact your GP to discuss the diabetes care available in your area;
- contact your local Community Health Council;
- contact the Diabetes UK or your local branch.

NATIONAL SERVICE FRAMEWORK FOR DIABETES: STANDARDS

Standard 1: Prevention of Type 2 diabetes

1. The NHS will develop, implement and monitor strategies to reduce the risk of developing Type 2 diabetes in the population as a whole and to reduce the inequalities in the risk of developing Type 2 diabetes.

Standard 2: Identification of people with diabetes

2. The NHS will develop, implement and monitor strategies to identify people who do not know they have diabetes.

Standard 3: Empowering people with diabetes

3. All children, young people and adults with diabetes will receive a service which encourages partnership in decision-making, supports them in managing their diabetes and helps them to adopt and maintain a healthy lifestyle. This will be reflected in an agreed and shared care plan in an appropriate format and language. Where appropriate, parents and carers should be fully engaged in this process.

Standard 4: Clinical care of adults with diabetes

4. All adults with diabetes will receive high-quality care throughout their lifetime, including support to optimize the control of their blood glucose, blood pressure and other risk factors for developing the complications of diabetes.

Standards 5 & 6: Clinical care of children and young people with diabetes

5. All children and young people with diabetes will receive consistently high-quality care and they, with their families and others involved in their day-to-day care, will be supported to optimize the control of their blood glucose and their physical, psychological, intellectual, educational and social development.

6. All young people with diabetes will experience a smooth transition of care from paediatric diabetes services to adult diabetes services, whether hospital or community-based, either directly or via a young people's clinic. The transition will be organized in partnership with each individual and at an age appropriate to and agreed with them.

Standard 7: Management of diabetic emergencies

7. The NHS will develop, implement and monitor agreed protocols for rapid and effective treatment of diabetic emergencies by appropriately trained healthcare professionals. Protocols will include the management of acute complications and procedures to minimize the risk of recurrence.

Standard 8: Care of people with diabetes during admission to hospital

8. All children, young people and adults with diabetes admitted to hospital, for whatever reason, will receive effective care of their diabetes. Wherever possible, they will continue to be involved in decisions concerning the management of their diabetes.

Standard 9: Diabetes and pregnancy

9. The NHS will develop, implement and monitor policies that seek to empower and support women with pre-existing diabetes and those who develop diabetes during pregnancy to optimize the outcomes of their pregnancy.

Standards 10, 11 & 12: Detection and management of long-term complications

10. All young people and adults with diabetes will receive regular surveillance for the long-term complications of diabetes.
11. The NHS will develop, implement and monitor agreed protocols and systems of care to ensure that all people who develop long-term complications of diabetes receive timely, appropriate and effective investigation and treatment to reduce their risk of disability and premature death.
12. All people with diabetes requiring multi-agency support will receive integrated health and social care.

Brittle diabetes

What is brittle diabetes and what treatment does it require?

The term brittle diabetes is applied to someone with Type 1 diabetes who oscillates from one extreme to another, i.e. swings from severe hyperglycaemia (blood glucose much too high) to severe hypoglycaemia (blood glucose much too low) with all the problems that are encountered with a hypo. Someone with this problem is frequently admitted to hospital for re-stabilization. The term brittle is not a good one because to some extent the blood glucose of all people taking insulin swings during the

24 hours from high to low and back again. It is therefore restricted to those people in whom the swings of blood glucose are sufficiently serious to cause inconvenience with or without admission to hospital.

It is important to realize that brittle diabetes is not a special type of diabetes and only applies when the instability is severe. This normally occurs at a time when perhaps someone may be emotionally unsettled. It is particularly common amongst teenagers, especially girls. It is most encouraging that, as emotional stability and maturity are reached, so brittle diabetes disappears, and most of these people will become reasonably stable and their frequent admissions to hospital will cease. During any particularly difficult period it is well worth remembering that it will not last for ever.

I have 'brittle diabetes' and my doctor has advised me to stop working. Am I entitled to any benefits?

The term brittle diabetes is used rather too loosely. It is usually taken to mean someone whose blood glucose rises or falls very quickly and who may develop unexpected hypos. Many conditions may contribute to this but one of the most common factors is an inappropriate dose of insulin. Other factors, which may contribute include irregular meals and lifestyle, poor injection technique, and general ignorance about the problems of balancing food, exercise and insulin. Few people have such difficulty in controlling their diabetes that they have to give up work, but welfare benefits are available to people with diabetes in the same way as they are to anyone else. There are some questions about Social Security benefits in Chapter 5.

5

Life with diabetes

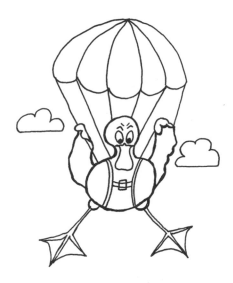

This chapter is meant to answer all the questions that affect daily living when you have diabetes. It covers a broad sweep from sport to holidays to surgical operations and illness. The section on *Other illnesses* should be read early on, so that you will know how to react if you are struck down by a bad attack of 'flu. All car drivers should read the section on *Driving*. At the end of the chapter is a miscellaneous section with questions that we could not find a place for elsewhere (e.g. electrolysis, ear piercing and identity bracelets). After reading this chapter, you will realize that there are very few activities that are barred to people with diabetes. Provided that you understand the condition, you should be able to do almost anything you wish.

Sports

My 13-year-old son is a keen footballer and has just developed diabetes. Will he be able to continue football and other sports? If so, what precautions should he take?

Your son can certainly keep on with his football. There is a very well known professional football player who has Type 1 diabetes so, if your son is good enough at the game, diabetes should not stop him becoming another great footballer. People with diabetes have reached the top in other sports, such as rugby, cricket, tennis, sailing, rowing, orienteering and mountaineering. Certainly all normal school sports should be encouraged.

There is, of course, the difficulty that the extra energy used in competitive sports increases the risk of a hypo. Your son should take some extra carbohydrate *before* a match or any other sports period – he could have a couple of sandwiches or biscuits or chocolate wafers. He will probably need another snack or maybe a sugary drink like fruit juice at half-time, and if possible should carry glucose tablets in his pocket.

He also needs to watch what he eats *after* the game has finished. The effect of exercise on the body can last well after the exercise has stopped (the muscles are restocking their energy stores with glycogen) and often blood glucose drops 2 or more hours after the exercise period. So he may need a snack then or, if he is due a meal anyway, he may need to eat slightly more than usual. It would also be a good idea to increase the usual bedtime snack if he has been exercising in the afternoon or evening. It's always best to monitor blood glucose levels in this situation.

Another way of preventing a hypo during exercise is to reduce the amount of insulin beforehand. So, if he is playing football in the morning, he could reduce his morning dose of quick-acting insulin by half. It takes trial and error to discover by exactly how much to reduce insulin for a given amount of exercise.

**I used to enjoy swimming, but have been worried about
going back to the pool since I have been on insulin. What
if I had a hypo?**

Whilst a hypo during athletics and most team games can be
inconvenient, a hypo while swimming can be more serious and
you are right to be concerned about it. However, don't let your
concern stop you swimming, just make sure that you are sensible
about it. There are certain simple rules that all people taking
insulin should follow before swimming – by following them you
can swim with complete safety:

- Never swim alone.
- Tell your companions (or teacher if you are still at school)
  to pull you out of the water if you behave oddly or are in
  difficulties.
- Keep glucose tablets on the side of the pool.
- Get out of the water immediately if you feel the first signs
  of a hypo.

If you are a keen swimmer and want to take up scuba diving,
then the British Sub-Aqua Club does impose some restrictions.
They require people taking insulin who wish to scuba dive to
have an annual medical review, not to have any long-term complications of diabetes, and insist that they always dive with another
person who does not have diabetes. You can contact the Club for
more details – the address is in Appendix 3.

Can I take part in all or any forms of sport?

The vast majority of sports are perfectly safe for people with diabetes. The problem lies in those sports where loss of control due
to a hypo could be dangerous, not only to you but to fellow participants or spectators. Swimming is an example of a potentially
dangerous sport but, if you take certain precautions (see previous question), it is safe to swim. However, in other sports (e.g.
motor racing), the risk of serious injury in the case of a hypo is
even greater. The governing bodies of such high-risk sports discourage people with diabetes from taking part. Discouragement

does not necessarily mean a total ban – the restrictions may vary depending on whether you are on diet, diet and tablets, or insulin. You can always contact the appropriate governing body and ask for their advice, and find out what (if any) restrictions they impose. Skiing is discussed in the section on *Holidays and travel* later in this chapter.

Are people with diabetes allowed to go parachuting? I want to do a sponsored parachute jump to raise money for charity.

You can probably do your sponsored jump, but it will depend on your current treatment. If you are on diet alone, or on diet and biguanides, restrictions are minimal. If you are on sulphonyl-ureas or insulin the restrictions are much greater – you will need a medical certificate to state that you are well controlled, and you will be permitted only to jump in tandem. The British Parachute Association (address in Appendix 3) can give you more information about this.

As a 30-year-old with Type 1 diabetes, can I join a keep fit class or do a work-out at home?

Yes, certainly. Keeping fit is important for everybody. Like everyone else, if you are unused to exercise, you should build up the exercises slowly week by week to avoid damaging muscles or tendons. Remember that exercise usually has the effect of lowering blood glucose, so you may need to reduce the insulin dose or take extra carbohydrate beforehand.

I have Type 2 diabetes and am overweight and not well controlled despite a maximum dose of tablets. I have been advised to join an exercise class. Will this be worth the effort?

People with Type 2 diabetes are usually overweight and do not take enough exercise. Lack of exercise is a risk factor for the development of Type 2 diabetes and vascular disease. It has been shown beyond doubt that, if you can change your lifestyle to include regular exercise and improve your fitness, this will have a major beneficial effect on your diabetic control and cardiac risk factors.

I take insulin and jog quite a bit. I would like to try running a marathon. Have you any advice on the subject?

Dawn Kenwright, who has Type 1 diabetes, is a long-distance runner at international level. Dawn resumed training within a few weeks of starting insulin and worked hard to discover by trial and error the effect of exercise/food/insulin on her blood glucose levels. Before running, Dawn has found that she needs plenty of 'slow' carbohydrate (in the form of porridge) to maintain her energy levels. During training sessions Dawn wears a bumbag containing glucose tablets and solution, but in competition she cuts back her insulin drastically and just carries glucose tablets. With careful preparation she rarely needs extra glucose. Dawn warns you to progress gradually from jogging up to a full marathon distance. She stresses that what is right for her will not necessarily suit everyone and makes the point that each athlete with diabetes has to work out their own solution for their particular sport.

Diabetes UK produces fact sheets on long distance running and some other sports. Once you have reached the required standard, you should think of joining Diabetes UK's team for the London Marathon.

Eating out

My wife and I entertain a great deal and we often go out for meals with friends or in a restaurant. I have recently been started on insulin for diabetes. How am I going to cope with eating out?

Nowadays people with diabetes usually eat similar food to anyone who is following a healthy lifestyle. Although you should normally try to avoid foods that are obviously high in sugar and fat, this may be difficult when you are visiting friends.

Restaurants or takeaways should pose less of a problem as you can select suitable dishes from the menu. Many people using a basal + bolus regimen choose to take extra short-acting insulin to cover the extra food they are eating.

People on two or more doses of insulin a day sometimes worry about how they are going to give their injections when they are away from home. Nowadays with insulin pens there should be no difficulty. If there is nowhere else to inject, you can always retire to the lavatory just before sitting down to eat! People who are less shy discreetly give themselves insulin into their abdomen whilst at the table waiting for the first course to arrive. The use of an insulin pen (see the section on *Insulin pens* in Chapter 3) can make the injection simpler, as bottles of insulin do not need to be carried around. Do not take your evening dose of insulin before leaving home in case the meal is delayed.

Fasting and diabetes

As a Muslim I wish to fast during Ramadan. Is this possible?

People with diabetes who fast during Ramadan may experience large swings in blood glucose levels, as a result of the long gaps between meals and the consumption of large quantities of carbo-hydrate-rich foods during the non-fasting hours. Therefore, if you have diabetes, you may be exempt from fasting. However, many people express a great desire to fast, and do not want their diabetes to prevent them from doing something they feel strongly about. If you have Type 2 diabetes and are treated by diet alone there should be no problem with fasting during Ramadan. However, there may be major changes in the type of food and drink that you consume during the non-fasting hours and this may affect your diabetes. If you are treated with insulin injections, sulphonylurea tablets, or a combination of the two, you should

Colour Plates Section

LIST OF PLATES

INSTRUCTIONS FOR USE

1 Remove the pen cap and unscrew the cartridge holder. Dial the return mechanism clockwise to ensure the piston rod is in its starting position. NEVER PUSH THE PISTON ROD BACK AS THIS MAY DAMAGE THE PEN.

2 Insert the cartridge into the holder - the coloured cap goes in first.

3 Screw both halves of the pen together firmly.

4 Cloudy insulins must be evenly mixed before injecting. Do not try to inject cloudy insulins if you can see the rubber piston in the small inspection window.

5 Screw a needle onto the end of the pen and remove the outer and inner caps. Remember to do an 'air-shot' before each injection.

6 Check the push button is fully depressed then dial the number of units you need to inject. Up to 70 units may be delivered as one dose.

7 Inject the insulin into your chosen injection site by pressing the push button fully home.

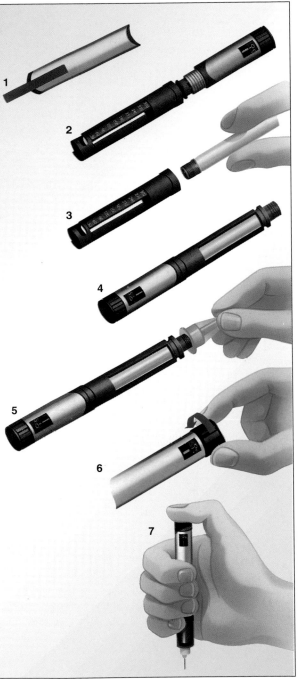

Plate 2   USING AN OPTIPEN

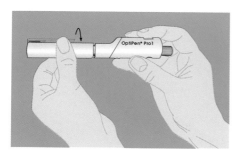

1   Twist off the pen cap.

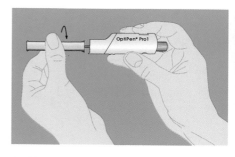

2   Unscrew the cartridge holder from the pen body.

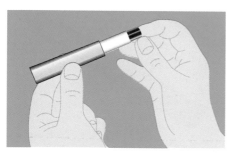

3   Put the insulin cartridge into the cartridge holder.

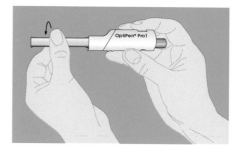

4   Peel off paper from the needle cap.

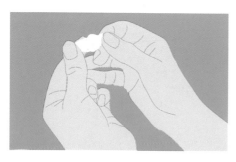

5   Screw the cartridge holder and pen body back together.

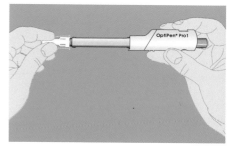

6   Peel off paper from the needle cap.

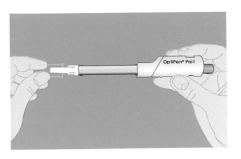

7   Put the needle onto the pen.

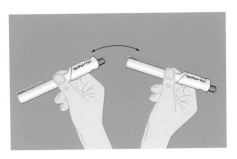

8   Remove the plastic cover from the needle.

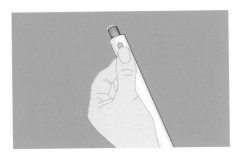

9   If your insulin is cloudy, gently turn the pen up and down until the insulin is mixed.

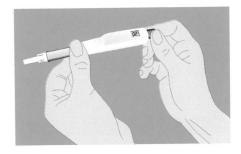

10 Press the safety button to release the dosage knob.

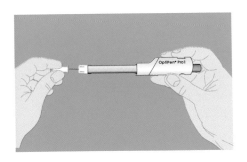

11 Take the lid off the needle.

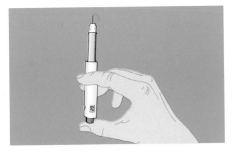

12 Press the dosage knob until it stays in and insulin should appear at the end of the needle. If insulin does not appear repeat steps 9–12.

(cont'd overleaf)

Plate 2   USING AN OPTIPEN (cont'd)

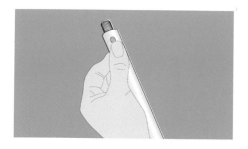

13 Dial up the dose you require.

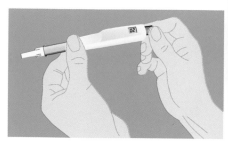

14 If you dial up too many units, simply turn the dosage knob backwards until your required dose appears on the display.

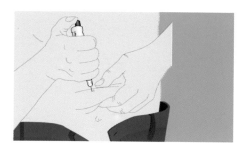

15 Inject insulin by pressing the dosage knob until it stays down. Leave the needle in skin for 10 seconds to allow your insulin dose to be fully completed.

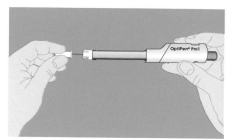

16 Remove the pen and replace needle cover and lid. The dosage given will stay on the display for 2 minutes.

CHANGING AN OPTIPEN INSULIN CARTRIDGE

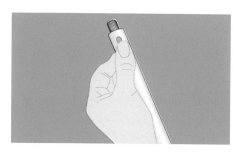

1 Press the safety button to release the dosage knob.

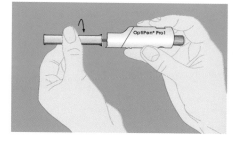

2 Unscrew the cartridge holder from the pen body.

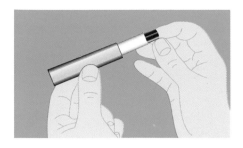

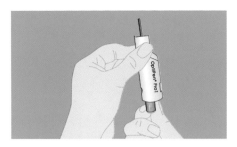

3 Remove the used insulin cartridge and put a new cartridge into cartridge holder.

4 Hold the pen as shown so metal plunger is pointing upwards.

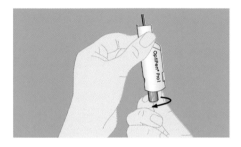

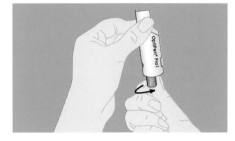

5 Turn the dosage knob to the left as far as it will go. The metal plunger will drop back into the pen body.

6 Then turn the dosage knob to the right as far as it will go. The metal plunger is now locked.

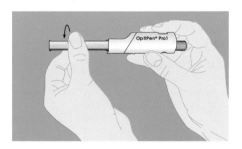

7 Screw the cartridge holder and pen body back together. Insert new needle. Your pen is ready to use. Perform a test shot first.

Plate 3   USING A BAYER ASCENSIA BREEZE

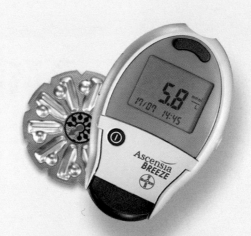

1 To open, hold the meter with the display screen down. Press on the back edge of the **'Open'** latch and pull up.

2 Insert the 10-test **Ascensia® AUTODISC.®** Keep the meter flat and snap it shut. The meter will automatically read the calibration information. No coding is required.

3 Pull and push the end tab to turn meter on and to automatically dispense a test strip. A blood drop icon flashes on screen to show the meter is ready to test.

4 Obtain a blood sample by pressing the lancing device firmly against the desired puncture site.

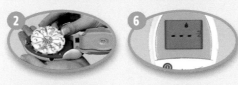

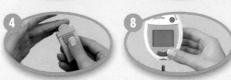

5 Touch the front edge of the **Ascensia® AUTODISC®** test strip to drop of blood until meter beeps. Blood is automatically pulled in to fill the test strip.

6 A sequence of dashes appear on screen while the meter calculates your blood glucose level.

7 After 30 seconds, your test result will be displayed on screen.

8 To discard the used test strip, hold meter with strip pointing down and press green release button. Press **'On/Off'** button to turn the meter off.

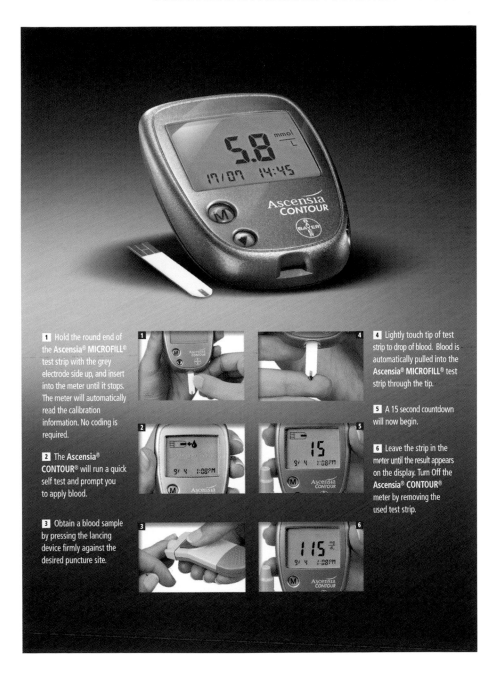

1 Hold the round end of the **Ascensia® MICROFILL®** test strip with the grey electrode side up, and insert into the meter until it stops. The meter will automatically read the calibration information. No coding is required.

2 The **Ascensia® CONTOUR®** will run a quick self test and prompt you to apply blood.

3 Obtain a blood sample by pressing the lancing device firmly against the desired puncture site.

4 Lightly touch tip of test strip to drop of blood. Blood is automatically pulled into the **Ascensia® MICROFILL®** test strip through the tip.

5 A 15 second countdown will now begin.

6 Leave the strip in the meter until the result appears on the display. Turn Off the **Ascensia® CONTOUR®** meter by removing the used test strip.

Plate 4   USING A LIFESCAN ONETOUCH ULTRA

ONETOUCH®
Ultra™
Created for hassle-free testing

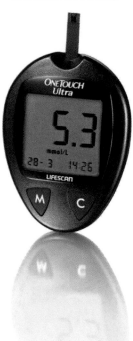

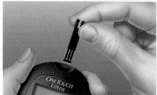

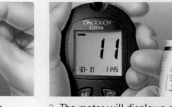

1. Always wash your hands thoroughly in warm water and then dry them on a clean towel before starting to test your blood glucose. Insert a test strip to turn the meter on. Contact bars to go in first.

2. The meter will display a code number. Ensure that this matches the code number on the test strip vial. If necessary, press the 'C' button to change the number. When the code numbers match, you may begin testing.

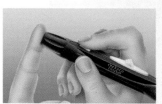

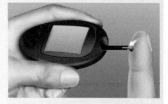

3. Hold the OneTouch® UltraSoft™ Adjustable Blood Sampler firmly against the side of your finger. Press the release button.

4. When the blood drop symbol is displayed, touch and hold the drop of blood to the top edge of the test strip where it meets the narrow channel.

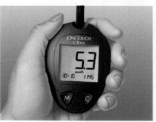

5. You will get the *test result in only 5 seconds* - the meter will count down from 5 to 1 and display the test result with date and time.

LIFESCAN
a Johnson-Johnson company

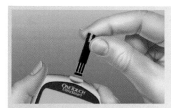

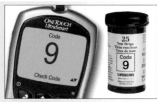

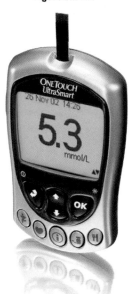

ONETOUCH®
UltraSmart™
The meter and electronic logbook in one

1. Insert a test strip, contact bars end facing up, into the meter test port.

2. Compare the code number on the display with the code number on the test strip vial. When the code numbers match, you may begin testing.

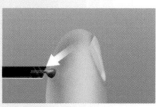

3. Hold the OneTouch® UltraSoft™ Adjustable Blood Sampler firmly against the side of your finger. Press the release button.

4. Touch and hold the drop of blood to the top edge of the test strip until the confirmation window is full.

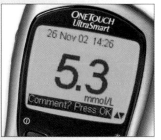

5. You will get the *test result in only 5 seconds* - the meter will count down from 5 to 1 and display the test result with date and time. Test results are automatically stored in the electronic logbook (memory).

6. You have the option to add a comment related to food, medication, health and exercise. Any comment you add goes straight to your logbook entry for that day.

Plate 5 SKIN LAYERS

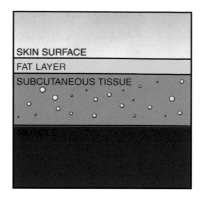

Choose an injection site where there is subcutaneous tissue. This type of tissue is located between the fat layer under the skin and the muscles which are below that.

discuss how fasting may affect your blood glucose control with your diabetes team, before Ramadan begins.

My local youth group is holding a sponsored fast over a weekend. I have Type 1 diabetes – can I take part?

It would be very difficult and perhaps dangerous for you to go without food and, even more important, drink, for 48 hours. The problem is that, even in the fasting state, you need small amounts of insulin to prevent the blood glucose rising. Having taken insulin, you would then need food to prevent an overshoot leading to a hypo. Anyone who goes without food for long periods produces ketones, which could be another hazard. While your friends are fasting, why not think up something else you could do safely to raise money, using some of your creative powers?

Holidays and travel

Do you have any simple rules for people with diabetes going abroad for holidays?

Here is a checklist of things to take with you:

- Insulin (or tablets)
- Syringes or insulin pen and needles
- Test strips (and finger pricker) and/or meter
- Identification bracelet/necklace/card
- Glucose tablets
- Starchy carbohydrate in case meals are delayed
- Glucagon
- Medical insurance
- Form E111 (from the DSS) if travelling inside the EU
- Hypostop Gel.

Each year on our summer holidays, our daughter becomes violently sick on the ferry. She recovers quite soon after we get back on dry land but she can keep nothing down during the crossing and it is very worrying.

We presume your daughter is on insulin and, as a general rule, people on insulin need hospital help once they start vomiting. Profuse vomiting leads to dehydration and if this is severe, the only treatment is a 'drip'. The other worry is the risk of a hypo if your daughter has already had her insulin. Don't be tempted to stop her insulin on the grounds that she is not eating.

There is no simple solution (apart from going by the Channel Tunnel) but the following ground rules may help.

- Take a standard antisickness tablet (e.g. Sea-Legs) at the recommended time before you sail.
- Try the 'acupuncture' wrist bands for seasickness now on sale at most chemists – they may just work for your daughter!
- Do frequent blood tests during the journey and immediately afterwards.
- If her blood glucose rises alarmingly, try giving her extra small doses of short-acting insulin.
- If her blood glucose values fall too low, give her Lucozade, Coca-Cola or some other non-diet soft drink.

Is it safe for someone with diabetes to take travel sickness tablets?

Travel sickness pills do not upset diabetes, although they may make you sleepy so be careful if you are driving. On the other hand, vomiting can upset diabetes so it is worthwhile trying to avoid travel sickness. If you do become sick, the usual rules apply. Continue to take your normal dose of insulin and take carbohydrate in some palatable liquid form, such as a sugary drink. Test your blood glucose regularly.

We are going on holiday and wish to take a supply of insulin and glucagon with us. How should I store them both for the journey and in the hotel?

Insulin is very stable and will keep for 1 month at room temperature in our temperate climate. However, it does not like extremes of temperature and can be damaged if kept too long at high temperatures or if frozen. It is best to carry your supplies in more than one piece of luggage in case one suitcase goes astray!

If you are travelling by air you should keep your insulin in your hand luggage – temperatures in the luggage hold of an aircraft usually fall below freezing and insulin left in luggage there could be damaged. Insulin manufacturers say it is stable for 1 month at 25° C (77° F), so it is perfectly safe to keep insulin with your luggage on the average holiday. Avoid the glove compartment or the boot of your car where very high temperatures can be reached. In tropical conditions your stock of insulin should be kept in the fridge.

Storage of glucagon is no problem as this comes as a powder with a vial of water for dilution. It is very stable and can survive extremes of heat and cold.

Airports now X-ray baggage for security reasons. Does this affect insulin?

Fortunately not.

I would like to go on a skiing holiday. Is it safe for me to ski, skate and toboggan? Should I take special precautions?

It is as safe for someone with diabetes to ski and enjoy other winter sports as it is for anyone else. Accidents do occur and it is essential to take out adequate insurance to cover all medical expenses. Read the small print in the insurance form carefully to ensure that it does not exclude pre-existing conditions like diabetes, or require them to be declared. In this case you should contact the insurance company and if necessary take out extra medical cover for your diabetes. Diabetes UK can provide travel insurance that will cover your diabetes (see Appendix 3). Physical activity increases the likelihood of hypos so always carry glucose and a snack as you may be delayed, especially if you are injured. Never go without a sensible companion who knows you have diabetes and understands what to do if you have a hypo.

Is sunbathing all right for people with diabetes?

Of course people with diabetes can sunbathe. Lying around doing nothing may put your blood glucose up a little, especially if you overeat as most people do on holiday. So keep up your usual tests as you may need extra insulin. On the other hand, increasing the temperature of the skin may speed up the absorption of the insulin and can lead to hypos, so be prepared for changes. Remember that sunbathing can increase the risk of skin cancer whether or not you have diabetes, so always take sensible precautions to avoid sunburn by covering up in the middle of the day particularly and using suncream with a high protection factor.

As I have diabetes should I be vaccinated when going abroad?

People with diabetes should have exactly the same vaccinations as anyone else. You are no more or less likely to contract illnesses abroad but, if you do become ill, the consequences could be more serious. In addition to the necessary vaccinations, it is very important to take protective tablets against malaria if you are going to a tropical area where this disease is found. More cases of this potentially serious disease are being seen in this country, usually in travellers recently returned from Africa or the East.

I am going to work in the Middle East for 6 months. What can I do if my insulin is not available in the country where I am working?

If you are working abroad for 6 months only, it should be quite easy to take enough insulin with you to last you this length of time. Stored in an ordinary fridge it should keep – but make sure that you are not supplied with insulin near the end of its shelf life. The expiry date is printed on each box of insulin.

Most types of insulin are available in the Middle East, but you may have to make do with a different brand name or even insulin from a different source (pig, cow or human). Strict Muslim countries regard pork and products from the pig as 'unclean' and porcine insulin may be hard to obtain in these countries. We have heard of customs officials in Saudi Arabia confiscating supplies of porcine insulin. To avoid this awkward situation it would be worth changing to human insulin before you try to enter such a country. The change may affect your control, and you should therefore make it in good time to allow yourself to stabilize before travelling. U100 insulin may be difficult to obtain outside the UK, USA, Australia, New Zealand, South Africa and parts of the Far East. Many European countries stock insulin in 40 units/ml only and special syringes for use with U40 insulin will have to be obtained. Diabetes UK can tell you which strength insulin is used in each country.

My husband has just been offered an excellent post in Uruguay, which he would love to accept. He is worried about my diabetes there and especially about the availability of my insulin. Can you let me know if my insulin can be sent by post?

It should be possible to obtain an equivalent type of insulin to your own in most parts of the world. If you are keen to keep up your normal supplies, Hypoguard Ltd are prepared to despatch syringes and equipment for testing blood and urine to all parts of the world. Unfortunately Hypoguard are not able to handle insulin. You might be able to make arrangements with a high street chemist who would be prepared to send insulin by post, or John Bell & Croyden in London will send insulin abroad. The address is in Appendix 3.

My friends and I are going to Spain to work next year. Can you tell me what I should take with me and whether I would have to pay if I needed to see a doctor?

Before you go abroad prepare yourself well – take spares of everything such as syringes, insulin, testing equipment and keep spare supplies separate from the main supply in case your luggage is lost.

Medical attention is free in all European Union countries, although you should obtain certificate number E111 (from your local Department of Social Security office) before you go. For longer stays abroad, you should contact the DSS. For countries outside the EU, you should insure your health before you go. Diabetes UK Careline can help you with this (see Chapter 11 for contact details).

I take insulin and need to fly to the USA. How do I cope with the changing time zones?

Flying from east to west (or vice versa) can be a bit confusing at the best of times and makes it difficult to know which meal you are eating. The box below gives some typical schedules for travelling from London to the east and west coasts of the USA plus the return trips. (If you use an insulin pen, the pattern for a basal + bolus regimen is exactly the same as the instructions here, apart from taking short-acting insulin before lunch on the plane. Many people using insulin pens are very used to injecting before each meal whatever time that is.)

When travelling keep to the following rules.

- Do not aim at perfect control. You have to be flexible especially on international flights. A hypo whilst travelling can be very inconvenient.
- Be prepared to check your blood glucose if you are at all worried and unsure how much insulin you need.
- In general, airlines are prepared to make special allowances for people with diabetes and cabin crew will do their best to help. Airlines say that they like to be warned in advance

1 London–New York

Get up as normal and have your usual dose of insulin and breakfast. The departure for New York is usually around 12.00 noon, so have a good snack before boarding the plane. During the flight you will be served lunch and an afternoon snack. You will arrive at about 2.00pm local time but your body thinks it is 7.00pm. Eat soon after arrival with your normal evening dose of insulin. If you then go to bed at 10.00pm local time (3.00am to you) you will need a small dose of long-acting insulin before a well-earned sleep.

2 New York–London

The problem here is that the flights are usually in the evening and the night seems to be very short. Assuming that you are going to try and sleep on the plane, you should reduce your evening dose of insulin by one-third and have this at about 6.00pm New York time followed by a reasonable meal. After take-off at 8.00pm you should be served with a meal and should then sleep. You will arrive at London at about 7.30am local time, although it will feel to you like 2.00am. Most people have another journey home, followed by a good meal and then a sleep. You should have a dose of long-acting insulin before this sleep and try and get back into phase by the evening (local time).

3 London–Los Angeles

This is an 11-hour flight usually leaving around midday and arriving on the west coast at 3.30pm local time which feels to you like 11.30pm. During this long flight you will have to have an injection of insulin on the plane and this is best if taken before dinner served at 6.00pm London time. It would be safest to give half your normal evening dose as short-acting insulin and then try and sleep. On arrival at the other side you will need to travel to your destination and will probably have an evening meal at what will feel to you like the early hours of the morning. A small dose of long-acting insulin before this meal would cover your subsequent sleep.

4 Los Angeles–London

Leave at 6.30pm and after a 10-hour flight you will arrive in London just after midday local time which will feel to you like 2.00am. Meals on this flight are usually served about an hour after take off and an hour before landing, in the hope that you have a good sleep between these two meals. One way round this arrangement would be to have a dose of insulin immediately before the first meal, giving a normal dose of short-acting insulin and half the normal dose of long-acting insulin. Immediately before the second meal you could have a small dose of short-acting insulin alone. This should last you through until the normal evening meal at your destination, which would be preceded by a routine evening insulin dose.

but in practice this should not be necessary. One of the problems of ordering a 'diabetic' meal is that it is often carbohydrate-free, so the standard airline meal might be more suitable.

Work

Can I undertake employment involving shift work?

Yes, certainly. Many people combine shift work with good control of their blood glucose. Shift work does, however, need a little extra care as most insulin regimens are designed round a 24-hour day. Shift workers usually complain that they are just settling into one routine when everything changes and they have to start again. It is hard to generalize about shift work as there are so many different patterns but, if you follow these rules, things should work out all right:

- Aim at an injection of short- and intermediate-acting insulin every 12–16 hours, or use a basal + bolus regimen. This way of giving insulin makes it much simpler to plan for shift work.
- Try to eat a good meal after each injection.
- Eat your normal snacks between meals every 3 hours or so, unless you are asleep.
- If there is a gap of 6 to 8 hours when you are changing from one shift to another, have some short-acting insulin on its own followed by a meal.
- Because your pattern of insulin and food is constantly changing, you will have to do more blood glucose measurements than normal, as you cannot assume that one day is very much like another.
- If your blood glucose results are not good, be prepared to make changes in your dose of insulin. You will soon know more about your diabetes than anyone else!

How can I cope with my diabetes if I work irregular hours as a sales rep?

Just as in shift work many people manage to combine an irregular lifestyle with good diabetes control. People who lead an erratic lifestyle usually find that the basal + bolus regimen gives them the freedom they require (there is a section on *Insulin pens* in Chapter 3).

If you have had an injection of insulin in the morning and normally have a fairly low blood glucose before lunch, then you will go hypo unless you eat at the right time. So a well-controlled person cannot afford the luxury of missing meals completely. However, it is always possible for you to have a few biscuits or even a sweet drink if you are getting past your normal eating time.

The occupational hazard of all sales reps, with diabetes or otherwise, is the mileage that they clock up each year on the roads. The dangers of hypoglycaemia while driving cannot be overemphasized and there is really no excuse for this now that instant blood glucose measurement is available.

Remember:

- If driving before a meal, check your blood glucose.
- If it is low, eat before driving.
- Always carry food in your car and have some immediately if you feel warning of a hypo.

Should I warn fellow employees that I might be subject to hypos?

Definitely. Hypos unfortunately can happen, especially when a person first starts using insulin. Warn your workmates that, if they find you acting in a peculiar way, they must get you to take some sugar. Warn them also that you may not be very cooperative at the time and may even resist their attempts to help you. Some people find it difficult to admit to their colleagues that they have diabetes but, if you keep it a secret, you run the risk of causing a scare by having a bad hypo and being taken to hospital by ambulance for treatment. A needless trip to hospital should be avoided.

My husband's hours of work can be very erratic. Sometimes he only gets 3 or 4 hours sleep instead of his normal 8 hours. Can you tell me what effect lack of sleep has on diabetes?

Lack of sleep in itself will not affect diabetes although, if your husband is under great pressure, his blood glucose may be affected. The real problem with working under a strain is the tendency to ignore diabetes completely and assume that it will look after itself. Unfortunately a few minutes of each day has to be spent checking blood glucose, eating a snack or giving insulin. These minutes are well spent.

I developed diabetes 5 months ago, 1 week after I had started a new job. I am coming to the end of my 6-month probation period and have been given two weeks' notice because of my diabetes. They said I could not do shift work because of my diabetes. Could you help?

This is a sad story and a good example of ignorant prejudice against people with diabetes. Of course there are many people on shift work who maintain good control – although it does require a bit of extra thought. You may well have a case under the Disability Discrimination Act and you should seek advice from your local Citizen's Advice Bureau.

I am a pub manager and have had diabetes for the past 19 years but my employers are now making me redundant. Apparently, their insurers cannot accept me for a permanent position owing to my diabetes. Who can help strengthen my case?

We know of several publicans with diabetes who run good pubs and still keep their diabetes under good control. However, people who work in licensed premises are at greater risk of drinking more alcohol than average and heavy drinkers are in danger from hypos (see the section on *Alcohol* later in this chapter). We wonder if you have been having frequent hypos, which has made it difficult to continue in your present occupation. Ask your clinic doctor and Diabetes UK to lobby on your behalf and seek legal advice from your local Citizen's Advice Bureau.

I have been refused a job with a large company because of my diabetes. Have I sufficient grounds to take proceedings against them for discrimination?

The Disability Discrimination Act covers people with diabetes but it can be difficult taking a company to court. We know this sort of discrimination does sometimes happen, especially in large organizations, although, of course, it is very difficult to prove. It may be possible for your case to go to an industrial tribunal to see if there are grounds for unfair dismissal but, as it sounds as if you have been refused a new job rather than dismissed from an existing job, then this could be difficult. The support of your own diabetes team will be important if you wish to take proceedings under the Disability Discrimination Act.

Diabetes UK has had discussions with medical officers responsible for occupational health in several large organizations. These have resulted in an employment handbook, which is circulated to diabetes clinics and occupational health doctors.

Other illnesses

I have recently had a severe cough and cold and have been given 'diabetic' cough medicine by the doctor. Since then my blood glucose has been very high. Could this be due to the medicine?

This is a good example of the effect that any infection or serious illness has on diabetes – it nearly always causes a rise in blood glucose. Unfortunately, many people often do not start to feel unwell until the glucose reaches danger level. People on insulin usually need more insulin when they are ill and yet they are sometimes advised to stop insulin completely if they do not feel like eating. This advice can be fatal. The rules when you are ill are as follows:

- Test blood/urine at least 4 times a day.
- If tests are high take extra doses of short-acting insulin.
- **Never** stop insulin.

It is of course possible to get over a bad cold by carrying on with your normal dose of insulin and accepting bad control for a few days. However, this means that your mouth and nose will be slightly dehydrated and it will take a few extra days before you feel back to normal. So you will probably feel better more quickly if you adjust your insulin and try to keep the blood glucose near normal.

Antibiotic syrup and cough linctus are often blamed for making diabetes worse during an illness such as 'flu or chest infection. In fact a dose of antibiotic syrup only contains about 5 g of sugar and is not going to make any real difference. It is the illness itself that unbalances the diabetes. In general, medication from your doctor will not upset your diabetes.

I have noticed that my son suffers from more colds since developing diabetes. Could this be due to his diabetes?

Many parents make this observation, but there is no real reason why the common cold should be more common in diabetes. However, a relatively minor cold may upset his diabetes control and lead to several days of illness (see previous answer). This may make it a more memorable event. To repeat the previous advice, never stop insulin.

My daughter keeps getting infections and has been rushed to hospital on several occasions with high ketones and requiring a drip. How can I prevent these infections? Will vitamins help?

It sounds as though your daughter has so-called 'brittle' diabetes and this must be very alarming for you. There are really two types of people with brittle diabetes. The first type includes those who are really very well controlled and can prove this by frequent blood glucose measurements below 7 mmol/litre and a normal HbA_{1c}, but who quickly become very ill and 'sugary' at the first sniff of a cold or the beginning of an infection. The other sort are those who are normally poorly controlled with blood glucose results all over the place and who therefore have no leeway when they become ill.

In the case of the first type it should be possible to increase the dose of insulin rapidly, giving extra doses every few hours depending on the blood glucose. The second type are more of a problem as it is the overall control that needs to be improved and this can be very difficult. Of course, if an infection (e.g. cystitis) starts off the trouble, this must be treated immediately with antibiotics. Provided that your daughter has a reasonable diet, vitamins will not help.

My 6-year-old daughter who is on insulin is troubled with frequent vomiting that occurs suddenly. She has ended up in hospital on several occasions as she becomes dehydrated. What can I do to avoid this?

Vomiting in a young child with diabetes has to be taken seriously and the hospital admissions are probably necessary to put fluid back into your daughter by means of a drip.

If the vomiting is associated with high blood glucose levels and ketones, then it may be possible to avoid these problems, if extra doses of short-acting insulin are given as soon as the blood glucose levels start to rise before vomiting occurs. As she gets older these attacks of sickness will improve.

What is the best treatment for someone suffering from hay fever? I understand that some products can cause drowsiness, which could affect my balance and be confused with a hypo.

You can use exactly the same treatment for your hay fever as people without diabetes, as it does not affect your control. Antihistamines are often used for hay fever and these may make you feel sleepy, but this should be easy to distinguish from a hypo. Remember that, if you are on antihistamines, you should take alcohol with great caution. Hay fever can also be alleviated by sniffing capsules, which reduce the sensitivity of the membranes in the nose.

I have just been in hospital with anaphylactic shock from a bee sting. I have diabetes controlled with tablets and wondered if this had anything to do with the severity of my reaction?

There is no connection between diabetes and allergy to bees.

What should I do if my son has an intercurrent illness while on tablets?

This can be a really difficult problem. Of course if your son is ill enough to need hospital admission, he will often be given insulin while his sugars are running high. At home, this is not as simple because there is no way of knowing what dose of insulin he may require, and an inadequate dose of insulin may even make matters worse. So, although in a perfect world he would have insulin for the duration of his illness, in reality it is acceptable for him to run high sugars for a day or so, in the expectation that they will soon settle down spontaneously. In a longer lasting illness, there is of course time to adjust the insulin dose in response to the results of blood glucose measurements.

What is the effect of other illnesses on diabetes? Is my son likely to suffer more illness than other children of his age?

Illnesses usually make diabetes worse in the sense that people on insulin need to increase the dose to keep blood glucose controlled. People on tablets or diet alone often find that a bad cold will upset their control. In the case of a prolonged illness or one needing hospital admission, a person with Type 2 diabetes may need to have insulin injections for a time.

Diabetes itself does not necessarily make people prone to other illnesses. In fact a survey in a large American company reveals that people with diabetes had no more absences from work than those without. Most children with diabetes grow up without any more illness than their friends.

Since I was diagnosed I have been very depressed. Is there any link between depression and diabetes?

People vary greatly in their mental response to developing diabetes. Some lucky ones accept their new condition easily, while others find the whole thing very depressing.

The depression seems to take two forms: at first, shock and even anger at the very onset, coupled with fear of injections and the unspoken fear of complications; a few weeks later comes the depressing realization that diabetes is for life, and not just a temporary disease that can be 'cured'. This type of depression seems to affect young people who are worried and are insecure about the future.

A few people with diabetes feel that, in some way, they are flawed, especially if they have previously been very body conscious. The best way round this feeling of inadequacy is to throw yourself into sporting activities with extra enthusiasm. Exercise is good for us all and people with diabetes have managed to reach the top in most forms of sport from ocean racing or rowing to international football.

If you treat your diabetes in a positive way rather than letting the condition control you, the depression will gradually lift.

However, if your low mood is interfering with your normal work and relationships, you should tell your GP about it.

How does stress and worry affect diabetes? I spend many hours studying and find that, if I study too long, I feel weak and shaky. Are there any side effects to pressure that may affect my diabetes?

In general, stress and worry tend to increase the blood glucose. A Scottish student told us that in the run up to her final examination, she had to double her insulin dose to keep perfect blood glucose control, even though she did not appear to be particularly anxious to her friends. Stress causes a release of adrenaline and other hormones, which antagonize the effect of insulin.

During periods of stress it may be difficult to keep to strict meal times, so you could be going hypo. You should check your blood glucose and, if it is not below normal, then you are simply experiencing the tiredness that we all feel after studying hard. Don't blame it on your diabetes but have an evening off from your studies.

Hospital operations

Recently, when I was in hospital to have my appendix removed, I was put on a 'sliding scale'. Please could you explain this, especially as it might save other people in a similar position from worrying?

We agree that the expression 'sliding scale' does sound rather alarming – but it is nothing to worry about. It can be difficult to predict exactly how much insulin someone will need during and after an operation. The way round this is to use a 'sliding scale' so that more insulin is given if the glucose in the blood is high. This is usually monitored every 1–4 hours and the insulin adjusted accordingly. Nowadays, during an operation, insulin is often given straight into a vein using a slow infusion pump. Most surgical wards have machines for measuring blood glucose and by doing this regularly the dose of insulin can be adjusted according to the result. In this way, diabetes control can be carefully regulated throughout the operation and until the person is eating again. At this stage the insulin may be given by 3 or 4 injections a day, the dose given at each injection being determined from the amount of insulin according to the 'sliding scale'.

Are there any problems with surgery for a child with diabetes?

Surgical operations on children usually involve a general anaesthetic and it is advisable to have nothing to eat or drink (nil by mouth) for 6 hours before the anaesthetic is given. Any difficulties caused by this period of fasting can be overcome by a glucose drip into the vein. The normal insulin injection is not given on the day of operation but small regular doses are either injected under the skin or pumped continuously into the vein. The dose of insulin is adjusted according to the blood glucose level. In minor operations where people are expected to be eating an hour or so later, these elaborate procedures may not be necessary and insulin may simply be delayed until the next meal is due. If an emergency operation is necessary, it is important that the doctors know that you have diabetes. This is another good reason for wearing an identification bracelet or necklace.

Must I tell my dentist that I have diabetes and will this affect my treatment in any way?

Having diabetes will not affect your dental treatment at all. However, it is important to remove all possibility of a hypo while you are in the dentist's chair. If you are on insulin, warn your dentist that you cannot run over a snack or mealtime. It is less embarrassing to mention this before the start of a session than to have to munch glucose tablets while the dentist is trying to administer treatment.

Obviously you must warn your dentist if he plans to give you any form of heavy sedation. If someone on insulin is to have dental treatment needing a general anaesthetic, this is usually done in hospital.

Is someone with diabetes more likely to suffer from tooth decay or gum trouble?

There is an increased risk of infection in people who are poorly controlled. The gums may become infected and this in turn may lead to tooth decay. However, someone who is well controlled is not prone to any particular dental problem – in fact, there is a positive advantage to avoiding sweets, which cause dental caries (tooth decay).

I have been told that, as I have diabetes, I don't have to pay for dental treatment. Is this true?

No. Dental treatment is not free to people who have diabetes. If you are entitled to benefits such as Income Support, you may be entitled to some help with the cost of treatment.

Driving

I drive a lot in my work and my lunch time varies from day to day. Does this matter? I am on two injections of insulin a day.

Yes, this can be a bit of a problem. The twice-daily insulin regimen is designed to provide a boost of insulin at midday to cope with the lunch time intake of food. Once the early morning injection of insulin has been given, there is no way of delaying the midday surge. It is very common for people who are well controlled on two injections a day to feel a little hypo before lunch. There are two possible solutions to your problem.

- Eat some biscuits or fruit while you are driving – only do this in emergencies as you will not know how much to have for lunch when you do get the chance to eat properly.

- Change your insulin regimen so that you have a small dose of short-acting insulin before each main meal and only have long-acting insulin in the evening to keep your diabetes under control during the night. You may have to eat snacks between meals but the three- or four-injection method should make the timing of meals more flexible. With an insulin pen an extra injection is really no hardship.

If I have diabetes, do I have to declare this when applying for a driving licence? If so, am I likely to be required to provide evidence as to fitness to drive?

Anyone whose diabetes is treated by diet alone does not need to inform the DVLA (Driving and Vehicle Licensing Agency). If your diabetes is treated by tablets or insulin, you must declare this when applying for a driving licence. If you already hold a driving licence, you must tell the DVLA as soon as you have been diagnosed.

When you have notified the DVLA, you will receive a form asking for details about your diabetes and the names of any doctors whom you see regularly. They will also ask you to sign a declaration allowing your doctors to disclose medical details about your condition. There is usually no difficulty over someone with diabetes obtaining a licence to drive.

If you are treated by tablets, you will be able to obtain an unrestricted licence, provided that you undertake to inform the DVLA of any change in your treatment or if you develop any complications of diabetes.

If you are treated by insulin, the licence will be valid for only 3 years instead of up to the age of 70, which is normal in the UK. It is the risk of sudden and severe hypoglycaemia, which makes people liable to this form of discrimination. In general the only people who have difficulty in obtaining a licence are those on insulin with very erratic control and a history of hypos causing unconsciousness. Once their condition has been controlled and severe hypos abolished, they can reapply for a licence with confidence. Diabetes UK has successfully campaigned for regulations on C1 licences to be changed. Previously, blanket restrictions were imposed on insulin users wishing to drive small vans and lorries between 3.5 and 7.5 tonnes. This now enables anyone on insulin, including those who have previously had their entitlement withdrawn, to be individually assessed on their fitness to drive. Restrictions on other Group 2 vehicles (heavier vehicles and passenger-carrying vehicles, such as mini-buses) remain. For more information, contact Diabetes UK.

When I was filling out a form for the DVLA, one of the questions asked whether I had had laser treatment in both eyes. Why do the DVLA need this information?

The DVLA may ask you to have a 'visual fields test' if you have had laser treatment in both eyes, and your licence will be revoked if you cannot pass this test. If you are having a visual fields test, we would recommend that you have the type in which both eyes are tested at the same time. This test, which examines both eyes together is the DVLA driving standard.

Do I have to inform my insurance company that I have diabetes?

When applying for motor insurance, you must declare that you have diabetes. Failure to disclose this can invalidate your cover if you need to put in a claim. The Disability Discrimination act 1996 has reduced the problems of insurers loading premiums surrounding motor insurance. The Act outlaws the charging of higher premiums for groups of people where no higher risk rate has been proven, as is the case with diabetes. Unfortunately, there are some companies that still discriminate, but Diabetes UK Services have arranged a car insurance scheme to help make life easier. (See Appendix 3 for more information.)

I have heard that a driver who had a motor accident while hypo was successfully prosecuted for driving under the influence of drugs and heavily fined. As someone who takes insulin I was horrified to hear this verdict.

Several people on insulin have been charged with this offence after a hypo at the wheel when the only 'drug' that they have used is insulin. It may seem very unfair but, for any victim of an accident, it is no consolation that the person responsible was hypo rather than being blind drunk. These cases emphasize the importance of taking driving seriously. Remember the rules:

- Always carry food/glucose in your car.
- If you feel at all hypo, stop your car (as soon as possible), take some glucose and move into the passenger seat.
- Check that your blood glucose is above 5 mmol/litre before driving again.
- On a long journey, check blood glucose levels every few hours.

I have been a bus driver for 15 years and was found to have diabetes 5 years ago. Up until now I have been on tablets but may need to go on to insulin. Does this mean I will lose my job?

As a bus driver you will hold a PCV (Passenger Carrying Vehicle) licence. People on insulin are not allowed to drive a PCV. You are faced with a very difficult choice – either to continue on tablets feeling unwell but holding down your job, or else to start insulin and feel much better, but lose your source of employment. We would have to advise you to go onto insulin as you will come to this eventually anyway.

Holders of a LGV (Large Goods Vehicle) licence will also lose their licence and thus their livelihood if insulin treatment is to be started. LGV drivers who have been on insulin *since before 1991 and held their HGV licence since then* may keep their licences provided that they can prove that their control of their diabetes is good and they are not subject to hypos.

I recently read a newspaper article that implied that people with diabetes who are breathalysed can produce a positive reading even though they have not been drinking alcohol. What does this mean?

Diabetes has no effect on breathalyser tests for alcohol even if acetone is present on the breath. However, the Lion Alcolmeter widely used by the police does also measure ketones, though this does not interfere with the alcohol measurement. Anyone breathalysed by the police may also be told that they have ketones and that they should consult their own doctor. These ketones may be caused either by diabetes that is out of control or by a long period of fasting.

Alcohol

My husband likes a pint of beer in the evening. He has now been found to have diabetes and has to stick to a diet. Does this mean he will have to give up drinking beer?

No. He can still drink beer but, if he is trying to lose weight, he will need to reduce his overall calorie intake and, unfortunately, all alcohol contains calories. There are about 180 calories in a pint of beer and this is equivalent to a large bread roll. Special 'diabetic' lager contains less carbohydrate but more alcohol so in the end it contains the same number of calories, with the drawback of being more expensive and more potent. He should probably also avoid the 'strong' brews, which are often labelled as being low in carbohydrate, as these are higher in alcohol and calories than the ordinary types of beer and lager. Low-alcohol and alcohol-free beers and lagers often contain a lot of sugar, so, if he decides to change to these, he should look for the ones also labelled as being low in sugar.

So overall your husband is probably better off drinking ordinary beer, but if he is overweight he should restrict the amount he drinks.

My teenage son has had diabetes since the age of 7. He is now beginning to show interest in going out with his friends in the evening. What advice can you give him about alcohol?

Most people with diabetes drink alcohol and it is perfectly safe for them to do so. However, if your son is on insulin he must be aware of certain problems that alcohol can cause – in particular alcohol can make hypos more serious. When someone goes hypo a number of hormones are produced that make the liver release glucose into the bloodstream. If that person has drunk some alcohol, even as little as 2 pints of beer or a double measure of spirits, the liver will not be able to release glucose and hypos will be more sudden and more severe.

In practice alcoholic drinks that also contain carbohydrate tend to increase the glucose in the blood. So the overall effect of a particular alcoholic drink depends on the proportions of alcohol to carbohydrate. For instance, lemonade shandy (high carbohydrate/low alcohol) will have a different effect on blood glucose from vodka and slimline tonic (low carbohydrate/high alcohol). Your son may notice that 'diabetic' lager is more likely than ordinary beer to cause a hypo because it contains less carbohydrate but more alcohol.

If your son has been drinking in the evening, then his blood glucose may drop in the early hours of the morning. To counteract this it would be sensible for him to eat a sandwich or cereal and milk to provide extra carbohydrate before going to bed.

I am 18 and go out a lot with my friends. I am careful never to drink and drive but, when it is not my turn to drive, I do drink quite a lot. I am careful not to miss any meals and I am not increasing my insulin as I used to when I first started drinking, but I have had quite a few bad hypos recently. Why should this happen?

This is because alcohol blocks the release of glucose from the liver (see the previous question for more information about this). If your blood glucose is dropping because it is a while since you have eaten or because you have been out and active longer than usual, then your body cannot come to the rescue as normal. Ideally it would be better if you could try not to have more than three or four units of alcohol in any one session. One unit of alcohol is half a pint of beer or lager or cider OR one glass of wine OR one single pub measure of spirits OR one measure of sherry or aperitif.

If you are going to have more than three or four units in one go, then make sure that you have your usual meal before you go out, have a snack while out and, very importantly, have a sandwich before you go to bed. Following this plan will help prevent you having hypos.

I believe that it is dangerous to drink alcohol if certain tablets are being taken. Does this apply to tablets used in diabetes?

In general the answer is no. Some people on chlorpropamide (Diabenese) experience an odd flushing sensation when they drink alcohol but those people can easily be changed on to an alternative tablet (e.g. gliclazide), which does not cause this problem.

The other consideration is that alcohol may alter the response to a hypo (this has been discussed in an earlier question in this section) and most tablets used for diabetes can cause hypos. If you are on tablets and are going to drink any alcohol, then you must be extra careful not to go hypo.

I've heard that there is evidence that a moderate amount of alcohol is part of a healthy diet, and that it reduces the risk of heart disease and strokes. My dietitian made me cut down my alcohol intake to one glass of wine a day, which is much less than I used to drink. What should I do?

Recent research shows that alcohol in moderation reduces the risk of heart attacks, strokes and premature death in people with diabetes (or without); indeed the effects may be even more impressive in people with diabetes. Our view is that moderate alcohol intake (up to a maximum of half a bottle of wine a day, or equivalent) should be encouraged, but within a calorie-regulated diet, if the person is overweight.

Drugs

My son was told that people with diabetes should not use Betnovate cream because it contains steroids. Is this true and why?

Most skin specialists avoid using powerful steroid creams such as Betnovate unless there is a serious skin condition. Very often a weak steroid preparation or some bland ointment is just as effective in clearing up mild patches of eczema and other rashes. Unfortunately too often the very strong steroids are often used first, instead of as a last resort. These strong steroids can be absorbed into the body through the skin and lead to a number of unwanted side effects. This advice applies to all people with skin problems and not just people with diabetes. One of the side effects of steroids is a rise in the blood glucose level. Thus, someone without diabetes may develop it while taking steroids and a person treated with diet only may need to go onto tablets or insulin.

If there are good medical reasons for your son to take steroids, in whatever form, he should be prepared to test his blood for signs of poor control. If he is already taking insulin, the dose may need to be increased.

Can you tell me if any vaccinations including BCG are dangerous for people with diabetes?

There is no reason why a child should not have full immunization against the usual diseases. Sometimes inoculation is followed by a mild 'flu-like illness, which may lead to a slight upset of diabetes control. This is no reason to avoid protecting your child against measles, whooping cough, etc. In some areas school children are given BCG as a protection against tuberculosis.

Children should also have the normal immunization procedures if they are travelling to exotic places (see the **Holidays** section earlier in this chapter).

My wife suffers from bad indigestion. She is afraid to take indigestion tablets in case they upset her diabetes. Can you advise her what to do?

Indigestion tablets and medicines do not upset diabetes.

Is it safe to take water tablets (diuretics) with diabetes?

Diuretics are given to people who are retaining too much fluid in the body. This fluid retention may happen in heart failure and cause swelling of the ankles or shortness of breath. Diuretics are usually very effective but, as a side effect, they may cause a slight increase in the blood glucose. This is especially true of the milder diuretics such as Navidrex, which belong to the thiazide group. The increase in glucose is only slight but can sometimes mean that someone controlled on diet alone may need to take tablets. People already on insulin are not affected by diuretics. The thiazide group of tablets is also used in the treatment of raised blood pressure.

Is there any special cough mixture for people with diabetes?

There are various sugar-free cough mixtures that can be bought from your chemist. However, there is only a tiny bit of sugar in a dose of ordinary cough mixture and this amount is not going to have any appreciable effect on the level of blood glucose.

I have been on insulin for diabetes for 7 years. I was recently found to have raised blood pressure and was given tablets, called beta-blockers, by my doctor. Since then I have had a bad hypo in which I collapsed without the normal warning signs of sweating, shaking, etc. Could the blood pressure tablets have caused this severe hypo?

Beta-blockers are widely used for the treatment of high blood pressure and certain heart conditions. They have an 'anti-adrenaline' effect, which theoretically could damp down the normal 'adrenaline' response to a hypo (there is a section on *Hypos* in Chapter 3). However, research has shown that beta-blockers do not reduce the adrenaline warning of a hypo. Some beta-blockers have been designed to have their effect only in the heart without blocking the general adrenaline reaction. These selective beta-blockers are theoretically safer for people taking insulin.

Please could you give me a list of tablets or medicines that may interfere with my diabetes?

The important medicines that affect diabetes have already been discussed in this section. There are no medicines that must never be used but the following might increase the blood glucose and upset your control:

- steroids (e.g. prednisolone, Betnovate ointment) and steroid inhalers (e.g. Becotide) – taken in tablet form may cause a rise in blood glucose level but inhalers or ointment will have this effect only in very large doses
- thiazide diuretics (e.g. Navidrex, Neo-Naclex)
- the contraceptive pill
- hormone replacement therapy (e.g. Harmogen, Prempac, Trisequens, Progynova)
- certain bronchodilators (e.g. Ventolin) – might have a slight effect on raising the blood glucose
- aspirin – in large doses might lower blood glucose
- growth hormone treatment.

Smoking

I am a 16-year-old on insulin. I would like to know whether smoking low tar cigarettes could interfere with my diabetes? Would it cause any restriction in my diet?

Smoking is unhealthy not only because it causes several cancers, particularly lung cancer, but because it leads to hardening of the arteries – affecting chiefly the heart, brain and legs. The proper advice to all people, especially teenagers, is not to smoke. Smoking will not directly affect your diabetes except, perhaps, by reducing your appetite.

When my doctor diagnosed diabetes, he told me to stop smoking. Could you tell me if there is a particular health hazard associated with smoking and diabetes? The problem is made worse for me by the fact that I have to lose weight and, if I stop smoking, I will do just the opposite.

Smoking is a danger, both to the lungs and because of the risk of increased arterial disease affecting any smoker. Someone who has long-standing diabetes is also at risk of problems with poor blood circulation, and it is foolish to double this risk by continuing to smoke. If the discovery that you have diabetes has come as an unpleasant surprise, this is a good time to turn over a new leaf and alter your lifestyle, by eating less and giving up cigarettes. It may be a lot to ask, but many people manage to carry out this 'double'. It will not kill you – on the contrary, you may live longer.

There is a lot of support available now for people who want to give up smoking, and your GP or practice nurse should be able to offer you advice on whom to contact. You may even find that they run an antismoking group or clinic. Some people find nicotine gum or patches useful, and we deal with these in a later question in this section.

Since my husband, who has had diabetes for 23 years, has stopped smoking, he has had high blood glucose tests. Why?

Your husband should be congratulated for giving up smoking. Most people who give up smoking put on weight, on average 4 kg (9 lb). This is because cigarettes suppress the appetite and make the body operate less efficiently, thus burning up more fuel (food). If your husband has put on weight, this explains his higher blood glucose levels. He should try to reduce weight to improve his diabetes. If he is already thin and his blood glucose levels are high then he will have to take tablets or insulin to get things under control.

My doctor has strongly advised me to give up smoking and suggested that I try nicotine patches. I was surprised to find that the information leaflet enclosed with the patches advised people with diabetes not to use the patches. Is this true?

It sounds as though the company are being overcautious. The main reason for giving up smoking is to reduce the damage that it does to the blood supply to the heart and legs. Each time someone has a cigarette, the nicotine that they inhale narrows the small blood vessels. This narrowing eventually becomes permanent, which explains why smoking increases the risk of such problems as heart attacks and gangrene. Nicotine patches have been shown to be a most effective way of helping people to stop smoking.

Nicotine has the same effect on the blood vessels whether from patches or from cigarettes. However, patches are no worse than cigarettes and, if they help you to give up smoking, the overall benefit will be enormous, especially with regard to your circulation. Don't be afraid to try nicotine patches in the recommended dose. The same advice applies to nicotine chewing gum and the newer nicotine inhaler.

Prescription charges and Social Security benefits

I believe that people with diabetes are entitled to free prescriptions. Please could you tell me how to apply?

One of the few definite advantages of having diabetes is exemption from payment on all prescription charges – even for treatment unconnected with the diabetes itself. People treated on diet alone are not exempt from prescription charges.

You must obtain a form, called *NHS prescriptions – how to get them free*, from a chemist, hospital pharmacy or a Post Office. Having filled in the form yourself, it must be signed by your family doctor or clinic doctor and sent to the local Family Practitioner Committee. The chemist should be able to give you the address. You will then receive an exemption certificate. Please remember to carry this certificate wherever you are likely to need a prescription, for example when going to the clinic or travelling in the UK. The certificate lasts for 5 years, and you will need to renew it at the end of that time.

To what Social Security benefits am I entitled now that I have diabetes?

There are no special benefits given automatically to people with diabetes. You may claim Disability Living Allowance if you have a child with diabetes who is under the age of 12, and it may be possible to obtain this allowance for a child up to the age of 16 if you can prove that the child needs extra supervision and care. Diabetes UK Careline can provide you with information to help you complete the necessary forms.

For more information about benefits, we suggest that you contact either Diabetes UK Careline, or the Disability Alliance (addresses in Appendix 3), or the Benefits Agency. The Benefits Agency is the organization that deals with Social Security benefits on behalf of the Department of Social Security, and you can make enquiries either at their offices or by phone. You will find their addresses and telephone numbers (they have several freephone enquiry lines) in your local phone book under 'Benefits Agency'.

Since developing diabetes I have found that my food bills have risen alarmingly. Are there any special allowances that I can claim to offset the very high cost of the food?

Most people with diabetes are not entitled to any special allowance and, indeed, there is no real need for them to eat different food from others. Special diabetic products are not necessary. Now people are encouraged to eat food that is high rather than low in carbohydrate, they do not have to fall back on expensive protein as a source of calories. There is a question in the *Diet* section of Chapter 2 offering suggestions on keeping down the cost of food.

My mother has had diabetes for 12 years and is subject to crashing hypos for no reason. She needs someone to be with her all the time. Would we be eligible for an Attendance Allowance as she needs watching 24 hours a day?

If you have to provide a continuous watch over your mother, then you would be able to apply for an Attendance Allowance. Before admitting defeat, however, it would be better to try every means to prevent the hypos. Presumably your mother is having insulin, though you do not mention the dose or type of insulin. It would be worth checking with the local diabetes service if anything could be done to reduce the frequency of hypos. Changing to more frequent but smaller doses of insulin might solve the problem. You may have to spend time and energy getting to grips with your mother's diabetes. It would do more for her self-confidence to abolish the hypos than to get an attendance allowance.

Miscellaneous

Is there any objection to my donating blood? I am on two injections of soluble insulin a day and my general health is fine.

There is no obvious reason why a fit person with diabetes should not be a blood donor. However, the blood transfusion authorities do not accept blood from people on insulin. They suggest that the antibodies to insulin found in all people having injections may, in some mysterious way, harm the recipient of the blood.

Is it true that someone with diabetes should not use an electric blanket?

It is perfectly safe for you to use an electric blanket, although most underblankets should be used only to warm up the bed in advance. The manufacturers usually recommend that underblankets should be switched off before you get into bed. However, there are now underblankets that can be left on all night on a very low heat and these would be safe to use, provided that you follow the manufacturer's instructions. Overblankets can be left on all night, but again you should always check the manufacturer's instructions.

Hot-water bottles are rather more dangerous as their temperature is not controlled. People with a slight degree of nerve damage can fail to realize that a bottle full of very hot water may be burning the skin of their feet. This is a recognized cause of foot ulcers. It is better to be safe than sorry and avoid the comfort of a hot-water bottle. Bedsocks are a possible alternative for cold feet, or you could try one of the small electric heating pads now on the market. Again you need to be careful how you use these and follow the manufacturer's instructions – not all of them are suitable for use in bed.

My 10-year-old daughter has had diabetes for 3 months. She has started to lose a lot of hair and now has a bald patch. Is this connected with her diabetes?

Yes, it could be. There are three ways in which diabetes and hair loss may be connected.

- If your child was very ill with ketoacidosis at the time of her diagnosis, this could lead to a heavy loss of hair. In this case, her hair will regrow over the next few months.
- Alopecia areata is a skin condition, which is slightly more common in people with diabetes. This is the likely diagnosis if your daughter has a well-defined bald patch with the rest of her hair remaining a normal thickness. If the patch is on the top of her head there is every chance that her hair will regrow over the next 6 months. There is no way of encouraging growth and steroid ointments may even cause permanent skin changes and make matters worse.
- Myxoedema or lack of thyroid hormones may occur with diabetes. If this is the cause of your daughter's hair loss, you will notice other symptoms such as mental slowing, weight increase and an inability to keep warm. All these symptoms can be corrected by taking thyroid tablets.

Shortage of body iron may also cause hair loss although this is not connected with diabetes.

I recently enquired about having electrolysis treatment for excess hair. I was told that, as I had diabetes, I would need a letter from my doctor stating that my diabetes did not encourage hair growth. Could I use wax hair removers instead?

There is no objection to you having electrolysis. Diabetes does not cause excessive hair growth. It sounds as though the firm doing the electrolysis is being overcautious.

Many women find wax hair removers useful for the less sensitive parts of the body. Make sure that the wax is not too hot.

Is it safe for people with diabetes to use sunbeds and saunas?

As safe as for those without diabetes. Exposure to ultraviolet radiation is known to increase the risk of skin cancer. Make sure that you can recognize a hypo when you are hot and sweaty. Keep some means of treating a hypo with you – not with your clothes in the changing room.

I have diabetes but would dearly love to have my ears pierced but, when I asked my doctor about this, he said there was a chance that my ears would swell. Please could you advise me if there is a great risk of this happening?

Anyone who has their ears pierced runs a small risk of infection until the wound heals completely. The risk in a well controlled person is no higher than normal. If your ears do become red, swollen and painful, you may need an antibiotic.

Is there any connection between vertigo and diabetes? I have had diabetes for just over 2 years controlled on diet alone.

Vertigo, in the strict medical sense, describes that awful feeling when the whole world seems to be spinning round. It is usually due to disease of the inner ear or of the part of the brain that controls balance. This is not connected with diabetes in any way. However, simple dizzy spells are a common problem with many possible causes, which may be difficult to diagnose. If dizziness occurs when you move from sitting down to the standing position, it may be the result of a sudden fall in blood pressure. This can sometimes be due to a loss of reflexes from diabetic neuropathy (see Chapter 9 on *Long-term complications* for more information about neuropathy). There are no other connections between diabetes and vertigo.

My husband's grandmother is 84 and has diabetes. Although she is fiercely independent, she cannot look after herself properly and will have to go into a residential home. Can you let me know of any homes that cater especially for people with diabetes?

Because diabetes becomes increasingly common in the elderly, most nurses in these homes are experienced in looking after diabetes. The staff of the home will probably be happy to do urine tests, ensure that diet is satisfactory and that she gets her tablets and, if necessary, insulin injections. If your grandmother-in-law is too fit and independent to accept a residential home, she may be a suitable candidate for a warden-controlled flat.

My wife, who developed diabetes a few weeks ago, is about to return to work. I feel that she should wear some sort of identity disc or bracelet showing that she has diabetes but she is reluctant to wear anything too eye-catching. Have you any suggestions?

It is very important that all people with diabetes, especially those on insulin, should wear some form of identification. Accidents can and do happen and it may be vital that any medical emergency team knows that your wife has diabetes.

Medic-Alert provide stainless steel bracelets or necklets which are functional if not very beautiful. They can also be obtained in silver, gold plate, and 9 carat gold. Medic-Alert's address is in Appendix 3.

SOS/Talisman (whose address is in Appendix 3) produces a medallion, which can be unscrewed to reveal identification and medical details. These can be bought in most jewellers and come in a wide range of styles and prices, including some in 9-carat gold. Other products are always coming on to the market, and *Balance*, the magazine produced by Diabetes UK usually carries advertisements.

Could you tell me what ointment to use for skin irritation?

The most common cause of skin irritation in people with diabetes is itching around the genital region (*pruritus vulvae*). The most important treatment is to eliminate glucose from the urine by controlling diabetes. However, the itching can be relieved temporarily by cream containing a fungicide (e.g. Nystatin).

I have recently been given a foot spa and was surprised to see a caution on the side of the box that it is not suitable for people with diabetes. Is this true?

If you have neuropathy (nerve damage), you should check with your diabetes team before using the spa. If you don't have neuropathy, make sure that you check the temperature of the water carefully and don't soak your feet for too long!

6

Sex, contraception and HRT

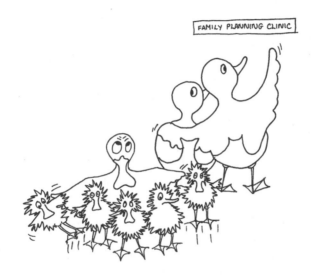

FAMILY PLANNING CLINIC

Although modern society has removed many of the taboos and inhibitions surrounding sex and contraception, many people still find it a difficult subject on which to ask personal questions. There are very many old wives' tales about diabetes and sex, and most of these are rubbish. Basically, people with diabetes are no different from people without diabetes in any aspect of sex, sexuality, fertility, infertility and contraception. There are, however, a few exceptions, such as the undoubted risk of impotence in men who have had diabetes for many years. In such people, there is usually evidence of neuropathy (nerve damage), although in some cases this is only mild. Even this has to be considered in relationship to the fact that impotence is a common problem in people without diabetes. There is certainly good evidence that women with diabetes are totally without risk of developing any problem analogous to impotence. Frigidity, on the other hand, is not uncommon in women, just as impotence is not uncommon in men, with and without diabetes.

Various contraceptive devices have at times been claimed to be less effective in women with diabetes – the evidence to support this is poor and, in our opinion, people with diabetes should consider themselves entirely normal as far as contraceptive practice is concerned.

There was, in the 1960s and 70s, much emphasis on the potential risk of precipitating diabetes when oral contraceptives were taken. It is now felt that the risks were grossly exaggerated in the media.

Impotence

I am male and have been diagnosed with diabetes. I have been told that diabetes could affect my sex life. Is this correct?

No. The vast majority of people, both male and female, are able to lead completely full and normal sex lives. This does not mean that problems do not occur but that most of these problems have nothing to do with diabetes. If, for any reason, diabetes control is lost with severe hyperglycaemia (high blood glucose), then this could affect your sex life. In a minority of people who have either severe nerve damage or arterial disease, a loss of sexual potency can be directly attributed to diabetes but this is uncommon. The majority of people, both male and female, can look forward to a completely normal sex life.

Is it normal for people with diabetes to suddenly find themselves totally uninterested in sexual intercourse? My husband is really upset about my lack of desire!

No more so than in people without diabetes. The feeling that you describe is more common in females than males, but no more common in those with diabetes than those without.

I have had erratic blood glucose levels recently. Would a low blood glucose affect my ability to achieve or maintain an erection and more importantly, my ability to ejaculate?

No, not unless the blood glucose is very low (less than 2 mmol/litre), in which case many aspects of nerve function are impaired; this could affect both your potency and ability to ejaculate. These will return to normal when your blood glucose is stable.

Am I likely to become impotent? I have had diabetes for 5 years.

There is no doubt that many people with diabetes worry about possible complications that may lie ahead of them at some stage in the future, and many men have loss of potency at the top of their worry list. Our advice is to worry more about keeping your diabetes under control and balanced and less about what future skeletons there might be in the cupboard. By ensuring that you have good control of your diabetes, you are doing everything that you possibly can to avoid trouble in the future, and the chances are that you will steer clear of difficulties throughout your life.

My husband, who is middle-aged with Type 1 diabetes, has been impotent for the past 2 years. Please will you explain his condition as I am worried that my teenage son, who also has diabetes, may also discover that he is impotent.

Impotence (or the fear of it) worries many people and is certainly not so rare that we can ignore it. It has been claimed that as many as 20% of males with diabetes (though the figure is probably not as high as this) may at some stage become impotent. Most impotent men are not suffering from diabetes: anxiety, depression, overwork, tiredness, stress, guilt, alcohol excess and grief can contribute to impotence. Any man may find that he is temporarily impotent and there is no reason why men with diabetes should not also experience this. Fear of failure can perpetuate the condition. Overwork or worry is frequently the cause of lack of interest in sex and even of impotence. Excess alcohol can cause prolonged lack of potency.

Some men with diabetes do become impotent, owing to problems with the blood supply or the nerve supply to the penis. This usually develops slowly and in the younger person we believe it can be prevented by strict blood glucose control. In the older person the condition does not usually respond well to treatment. In this age group impotence is more commonly due to other factors and not to diabetes. We hope that you will be encouraged to discuss the matter further with your own doctor or with the doctor at the diabetes clinic.

My wife left me because I was impotent and the doctors say that there is nothing they can do for me – why was I not told about any treatments available?

We are surprised that the doctors said that there is nothing they can do for you, because, even for those who are completely impotent, there are now several treatments that can be tried. There are questions about treatments for impotence later in this section.

It must be very upsetting to think that your marriage broke up on account of your impotence. In our experience, most wives are sympathetic and understanding about impotence (whatever the cause) provided that both partners can talk about the matter in an open manner. We have known frank discussions leading to an increase of affection within marriage. Keeping things bottled up leads to the aggression and resentment that emerges from your question.

Recently, I have had trouble keeping an erection – has this anything to do with my diabetes? I also had a vasectomy a few years ago.

This is difficult to answer without knowing more about you and your medical history. Certainly it is unlikely that the vasectomy had anything to do with your current problem. Failure to maintain an adequate erection may occasionally be an early symptom of diabetic neuropathy. However, and at least as commonly, it is often a symptom of overwork or simply growing older and you would need detailed tests to be sure of the cause.

I suffered a stroke affecting the right side of my body 12 months ago at the age of 40 and now suffer from partial impotence. The onset seemed to coincide not with the stroke but with taking anticoagulants. Are these known to cause impotence? I have heard that blood pressure tablets can cause impotence and I have been taking these for 3 months and wonder whether this is a factor?

A severe stroke can sometimes be associated with impotence. A stroke is often due to narrowing of the arteries inside the head: the arteries elsewhere may also be narrowed and, if those supplying blood to the penis are affected, it could contribute to your impotence. You are also quite right about the question of drugs. Some blood pressure lowering drugs may cause impotence and can interfere with ejaculation. It would be unwise to stop taking the drugs since this would lead to loss of control of your blood pressure without first asking your doctor to try you on different tablets for your high blood pressure to see if this helps. Anticoagulant tablets are not known to cause impotence.

I have been impotent for months. Is there some drug or hormone that will help me?

It is extremely rare that impotence is due to a hormonal abnormality. Many cases of impotence are due to psychological causes and often respond to appropriate advice and occasionally drug treatment. If you have a hormonal defect, treatment with replacement hormones (testosterone) will cure that particular form of impotence. It is essential to get a correct diagnosis in order to ensure appropriate therapy. It has been shown that the injection of a drug called papaverine directly into the penis can sometimes be helpful. It leads to an erection and, in people who have become impotent, the result is often good enough to make this an acceptable and effective form of therapy.

Viagra (sildenafil) is the first oral treatment for impotence to be licensed in the UK. It works by helping to relax the blood vessels in the penis, allowing blood to flow into the penis causing an erection. It will only help a man to get an erection if he is sexually stimulated. It is available to men with diabetes on the NHS, but officially the amount is limited to 4 tablets a month. It is important to use the full strength (100 mg) as lower amounts are less likely to have the desired effect.

I have used Viagra for 3 years for impotence. At first it worked very well but the effect now seems to be wearing off. Is there anything else I can try?

Recently another drug has come onto the market, which is designed to help people improve their erections. It is called apomorphine (or Uprima), and should be placed under the tongue about 20 minutes before you want sex. Apomorphine has about the same success rate as Viagra, but may help some people who do not respond to Viagra. The starting dose of apomorphine is 2 mg but, if this is no help, you can try a 3 mg dose. Apomorphine seems to be a safe drug, but you should avoid it if you have severe heart problems or if your blood pressure is low. You should wait 8 hours before repeating the dose of apomorphine.

Is there any other treatment for impotence apart from Viagra?

Yes. Depending on the cause, there are several effective forms of therapy. Counselling by a therapist trained in this subject can be helpful, particularly in cases where the stresses and conflicts of life are the root cause. Testosterone is effective in those with a hormone deficiency. Vacuum therapy, with a device that looks like a rigid condom, is also a another (if expensive) form of therapy, which has been useful in many cases. Injections of papaverine or alprostadil into the penis, and penile implants (which require an operation) are also effective. The best choice for an individual requires a considerable amount of thought and discussion with your doctor. Many diabetes clinics hold special clinics for treatment of impotence.

After sexual intercourse I recently suffered quite a bad hypo. Is this likely to happen again and if so, what can be done to prevent it?

This form of physical activity can, like any other, lower the blood glucose level and lead to hypoglycaemia. When this happens, and it is not at all uncommon, then the usual remedies need to be taken – more food or sugar beforehand or immediately afterwards. You may find it useful to keep some quick-acting carbohydrate close at hand, perhaps on a bedside table.

Contraception and vasectomy

I have diabetes and want to start on the Pill. Are there any extra risks that women with diabetes run in using it?

Use of the oral contraceptive pill is the same in both women with diabetes and women without diabetes. It is now well known that the pill carries with it small risks of rare conditions such as venous thrombosis (where a vein becomes blocked by a blood clot) and pulmonary embolus (where an artery in the lung becomes blocked by a blood clot), as well as occasionally high blood pressure, although these risks are obviously less than those of pregnancy itself. This is why all women should be examined and questioned before starting the pill because there are a few conditions where it is best avoided and other methods of contraception used. The same arguments apply equally to women with and without diabetes. Healthy women with diabetes who have been checked the same way as those without diabetes may certainly use the pill and there are no additional risks.

When women with diabetes start using the pill there is sometimes a slight deterioration of control. This is rarely a problem and is usually easily dealt with by a small increase in treatment, which in those taking insulin may mean a small increase in the dose. It is a simple matter to monitor the blood or urine level and make appropriate adjustments.

There is nothing to suggest that the pill causes diabetes. It is all right for the relatives of people with diabetes to use the pill but of course they, like others, should attend for regular checks by their general practitioner or family planning clinic.

My doctor prescribed the pill for me but on the packet it states that they are unsuitable for people with diabetes. As my doctor knows that I have diabetes is it safe enough for me?

Yes. There used to be some confusion about whether the pill was suitable for women with diabetes but there is now general agreement that they may use the pill for contraceptive purposes without any increased risks compared with those who do not have diabetes.

I want to try the progesterone-only contraceptive pill. Is it suitable for women with diabetes?

Yes, although recently these have become less popular for all women.

I have just started the menopause and wondered if I have to wait two years after my last period before doing away with contraception?

Although periods may become irregular and infrequent at the start of the menopause, it is still possible to be fertile, and this advice is a precaution against unwanted pregnancy. It applies equally to women with diabetes as to those who do not.

I have diabetes and I am marrying a man with diabetes in 8 weeks' time. Please could you advise me on how to stop becoming pregnant?

We are not quite clear whether you wish to be sterilized and not have children at all or whether you are just seeking contraceptive advice. If you and your fiancé have decided that you do not want to have the anxiety of your children inheriting diabetes and have made a clear decision not to have children, you have the option of your fiancé having a vasectomy or being sterilized yourself.

These are very fundamental decisions and will require careful thought because they are probably best considered as irreversible procedures. If you are quite certain about not having children, one of you having a sterilization would be the best plan. We would advise you both to discuss this with your GP and seek referral either to a surgeon for vasectomy for your fiancé or to a gynaecologist for sterilization. Whichever you decide, you must both attend since no surgeon will undertake this procedure unless he is convinced that you have thought about it carefully and have come to a clear, informed decision.

If our interpretation of your question has not been right and you are merely looking for contraceptive advice, then the best source of this is either your GP or the local family planning clinic. All the usual forms of contraceptives are suitable for women with diabetes, so it is just a question of discovering which best suits you and your partner.

Can you please give me any information regarding vasectomy and any side effects it may have for men with diabetes?

Vasectomy is a relatively minor surgical procedure, which involves cutting and tying off the vas deferens – the tube that carries sperm from the testes to the penis. Vasectomy may be carried out under either local or general anaesthesia usually as a day case. It would be simpler to have it under local anaesthesia as this will not disturb the balance of your diabetes. Side effects of the operation are primarily discomfort although infections and complications do rarely occur.

There are a few medical reasons for avoiding this operation but they apply equally to men without diabetes as they do to men with diabetes and your doctor will be able to discuss these with you.

I have been warned that IUDs are more unreliable in women with diabetes. Is this really true?

IUDs (intrauterine contraceptive devices) are generally regarded as slightly less reliable contraceptives than the pill, and there has been one report suggesting they may be even less reliable when used by women with diabetes. Not all experts agree about this, as there are no other reports confirming this observation. There has also been a report suggesting that women with diabetes may be slightly more susceptible to pelvic infections when using an IUD. On balance, our recommendation is that IUDs should be considered as effective and useful in women with diabetes as in those who do not have diabetes.

Thrush

I keep getting recurrence of vaginal thrush and my doctor says that, as I have diabetes, there is nothing that I can do about this – is this correct?

Thrush is due to an infection with a yeast that thrives in the presence of a lot of glucose. If your diabetes is badly controlled and you are passing a lot of glucose in your urine, you will be very susceptible to vaginal thrush and, however much ointment and cream you use, it is likely to recur. The best line of treatment is to control your diabetes so well that there is no glucose in your urine, and then the thrush will disappear, probably without the need for any antifungal treatments, although these will speed the healing process. As long as you keep your urine free from glucose you should stay free from any recurrence of the thrush.

I suffer with thrush. My diabetes has been well controlled for 10 years now. I do regular blood tests and most of them are less than 10 mmol/litre and, whenever I check a urine test, it is always negative. I have been taking the

oral contraceptive pill for 3 years and I understand that both diabetes and the pill can lead to thrush. Can you advise me what to do?

Since your diabetes is well controlled and your urine consistently free from glucose, diabetes can probably be excluded as a cause of the thrush. One has to presume that in your case you are either being reinfected by your partner or that it is a relatively rare side effect of the pill, and you would be best advised to seek alternative forms of contraception.

Hormone replacement therapy (HRT)

Can you tell me if hormone replacement therapy for the menopause is suitable for people with diabetes?

Hormone replacement therapy (HRT) for the menopause consists of small doses of oestrogen and progesterone given to replace the hormones normally produced by the ovaries. Oestrogen levels in the blood at this time begin to decline and, if they decline rapidly, they can cause unpleasant symptoms, such as hot flushes. Replacement therapy is thus designed to allow a more gradual decline in circulating hormones. Hormone replacement therapy is not usually advised in people with certain conditions such as stroke, thrombosis, high blood pressure, liver disease or gallstones. HRT may have a slight worsening effect on diabetes similar to the contraceptive pill (as we have discussed earlier in this chapter). Some doctors are reluctant to give HRT to any woman and may use diabetes as an excuse for not prescribing it. However, small doses of female hormones can cause dramatic relief of menopausal symptoms and there is no reason why you should not benefit from them provided that you have no history of stroke, thrombosis, etc.

There is good evidence that HRT reduces both osteoporosis and possibly vascular disease in postmenopausal women. The benefits probably outweigh the risks.

I want to try and avoid osteoporosis by taking HRT. As I have diabetes, is this sensible?

Yes. See the question above for our answers on taking HRT generally.

Are the patch forms of HRT as suitable for women with diabetes as the tablets?

Yes.

During the past 5 years I have had trouble with my periods being very heavy and on several occasions I have become very anaemic. I have tried HRT, which interferes with control of my diabetes, and it has been suggested that I have a hysterectomy. I have heard that depression is common after this operation and that HRT is often given to alleviate this feeling but, if this treatment makes my control more difficult, how will I cope?

Many people do have the impression that depression is common following hysterectomy. There is no reason for this. Anyone might get depressed after an operation in the same way that they would after any illness. A few women may feel that, if they have their womb removed, they have lost some of their femininity and therefore will become depressed. However, the womb is merely a muscle and has no effect at all on feminine characteristics apart from its relationship with menstruation. Unless the ovaries are taken out at the same time, there is no reason why you should require HRT. If the ovaries are removed, then HRT should not then upset your diabetes as you will be taking it to replace the hormones that you were producing yourself before the operation. The best person to discuss this with is your doctor.

Termination of pregnancy

I have become pregnant and really don't want a baby at the moment. Is diabetes grounds for termination of pregnancy?

No, not unless your doctor considers that the pregnancy would be detrimental to your health, which may occasionally be the case. All the reasons for termination of pregnancy apply equally to people without diabetes as to people with diabetes.

I am going into hospital for an abortion. I am worried that the doctors might not do it as I have diabetes. Should I have told someone?

There is no added hazard for women with diabetes who undergo termination of pregnancy, and care of the diabetes during this operation does not raise any special difficulties but it is still a good idea to tell your gynaecologist.

Infertility

I have recently got married and my wife and I are keen to start a family. Are people with diabetes more likely to be infertile than those who do not have diabetes?

There is nothing to suggest that men with diabetes are any less fertile than men who do not have diabetes and this is generally true also for women. In the case of women, however, extremely poor diabetes control with consistently high blood glucose readings is associated with reduced fertility. This is probably just as well as there is good evidence to show that the outcome of pregnancy is much worse in women who conceive when their control is poor.

I have been trying for a baby for years and we have now decided to go for fertility counselling and possible treatment. Can people with diabetes expect the same treatment for infertility as people without?

Yes. As mentioned in the previous question, diabetes is rarely the cause of infertility. If control is anything other than excellent, then improving control should be the first goal. If that is not successful than expert opinion on management from a specialist is the next step.

7
Pregnancy

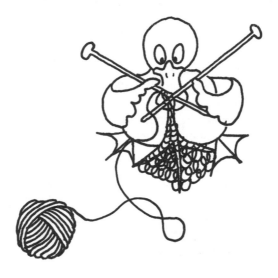

Pregnancy was the first aspect of life with diabetes where it was shown without any doubt that poor blood glucose control was associated with many complications for both mother and child, and that these complications were avoidable by strict control. The outcome for women with diabetes who are pregnant and for the babies that they carry is directly related to how successful these mothers are in controlling their blood glucose concentration. If control is perfect from the moment of conception to delivery, then the risks of pregnancy to mother and baby are little greater than in women without diabetes.

We now know that poor control when the egg is fertilized (conception) can affect the way in which the egg divides and changes into the fetus (in which all organs and limbs are present but very small) in such a way as to cause congenital abnormalities (such as harelip, absence of the bone at the base of the spine, and holes in the heart). The risk of this happening can be reduced to a minimum, and possibly even eliminated, by ensuring perfect control (normal HbA_{1c}) before you become pregnant.

For women who become pregnant when their control is poor, there will be an increased risk of congenital abnormalities in their babies – some of which may be detectable by ultrasound very early in pregnancy, when termination is possible, if a major defect is found. When no defect is detected, the outcome of the pregnancy will still be dictated by the mother's degree of control during her 40 weeks of pregnancy and during labour and delivery. Modern antenatal care is usually shared between the diabetes specialist and the obstetrician, often at a joint clinic. So long as control remains perfect (normal HbA_{1c}) and pregnancy progresses normally, there is no need for hospital admission. With the excellent control that is now possible, the baby will develop normally and we believe that the pregnancy can be allowed to go to its natural term (40 weeks). If spontaneous labour begins, the procedure is no different from that for a woman without diabetes, other than the continued need to keep the mother's blood glucose normal to prevent hypoglycaemia in the infant shortly after birth.

Women with diabetes are not immune to obstetric and antenatal complications and these will be treated in the same way as they would be in women without diabetes. If a woman cannot achieve satisfactory control of her diabetes at home, then her admission to hospital becomes essential, but there are very few mothers who cannot achieve and maintain normal blood glucose values as an outpatient, at least while they are pregnant. It is a remarkable example of the importance of motivation in the struggle for good diabetes control. The single-mindedness of a pregnant woman makes her able to cope with almost anything to protect her growing baby from harm. Sadly this motivation is often lost once the pregnancy is over and control slips back to where it was before.

A very comprehensive pregnancy magazine is available from Diabetes UK.

Prepregnancy

The man I am going to marry has diabetes. Will there be any risk of any children we have in having diabetes?

If you do not have diabetes yourself and there is no diabetes in your family, then the risk of your children developing diabetes in childhood or adolescence, if their father has diabetes, is probably about 1 in 20. Provided that you are both in good health it is certainly all right to have a family. If you and your fiancé both had Type 1 diabetes, then there would be an even greater risk of your children developing diabetes.

There is a rare form of Type 2 diabetes in which there is a strong hereditary tendency. This is called maturity onset diabetes of the young, commonly known as MODY. Were you or your fiancé to have this, the risk of your children getting diabetes of this unusual kind would then be rather high. It is often a relatively mild form of diabetes and runs true to type throughout the generations.

The study of inheritance of diabetes is a complicated subject and you would be well advised to discuss this further with your specialist or a professional genetic counsellor.

I am worried that, if I become pregnant whilst my husband's diabetes is uncontrolled, the child will suffer – am I right?

No. There is no known way in which poor control of your husband's diabetes can affect the development of your child.

I am 25 years old and have Type 1 diabetes. My husband and I plan to start a family but first I would like to complete a 3 year degree course at university. By the time this course finishes I will be 29. Can you tell me if I shall then be too old to have a baby?

You pose a difficult question as to the ideal age at which someone with diabetes should have a baby. The age of 29 is not too old to start a family but there are certain advantages in starting younger, particularly if you have diabetes and if you plan more than one pregnancy. Starting a family may be hard work whether you have diabetes or not. If you add increasing age to the difficulties, we are sure that you will understand why it is normally recommended starting earlier rather than later. It is difficult to give exact personal advice to individual people and the right person to talk to is your clinic doctor who knows both you and your diabetes.

I have diabetes treated by tablets, which I chose to take rather than insulin, and I want to become pregnant again. As I have had a previous miscarriage, I am worried about the chance of this recurring. Both my husband and I smoke a lot. How can I make sure that this pregnancy is successful?

Your control of your diabetes will certainly affect the outcome of your pregnancy – better control leads to more successful pregnancies. As you are planning your pregnancy, you can make sure that you establish good control before conception. Your control is probably best maintained by either diet alone or, if this fails, by diet with insulin. We do not advise women to take tablets throughout pregnancy, although they do not harm the baby if they are taken inadvertently in the early part of pregnancy. The tablets can cross into the baby's circulation and stimulate insulin secretion from the pancreas causing hypoglycaemia in the baby shortly after birth.

It should also be said here that most women of childbearing age are already being treated with insulin, so they are not normally faced with your decisions.

You obviously know already that smoking affects the baby and that heavy smoking is associated with more miscarriages and smaller babies. In asking the question we suspect that you already know the answer – take insulin and give up smoking.

There is also more recent evidence to link even modest regular alcohol intake in pregnancy with an unfavourable outcome as far as the baby is concerned, so we suggest that you should stop drinking alcohol until the pregnancy is over.

Why must I ensure that my diabetes control is perfect during pregnancy?

This is to ensure that you reduce the risks to yourself and your baby to an absolute minimum. If you are able to achieve this degree of control from before the time of conception through to the time of delivery, you can reduce the risks to your baby and these risks will be virtually indistinguishable from those to babies born to women without diabetes. On the other hand, if you do not control your diabetes properly and pay no attention to it, then the risk to your baby increases dramatically.

Pregnancy management

When I was 7 months pregnant, I developed diabetes. I had 8 units of insulin a day. After my baby was born, the tests were normal so I stopped taking insulin. I would now like another baby. My GP says I could develop permanent diabetes. Another doctor, however, says this is very unlikely – please could you advise me?

You have had what we call gestational diabetes (i.e. diabetes that occurs during pregnancy and then goes away again when you are not pregnant). The chances are that this will recur in all your subsequent pregnancies. You may well find that at some stage it does not get better at the end of the pregnancy and that you then have permanent diabetes. Even if you do not have further pregnancies, you are a 'high risk' (greater than 1 in 2) case for developing diabetes at some stage in the future. Your pancreas produces enough insulin to cope with everyday life but the extra demands of pregnancy are more than it can manage, hence the need for extra insulin. You should pay particular attention to your diet and fitness, and keep your weight at even slightly below your ideal weight for your height. The decision about further pregnancies with the greater risk of developing permanent diabetes is one that you and your partner must make after you understand the facts.

When I had my first baby, I was in hospital for the last 2 months and I was given a caesarean section after 36 weeks of pregnancy. My baby weighed 3.7 kg (8 lb 4 oz) even though it was 4 weeks early. During my most recent pregnancy I was allowed to go into labour at 39 weeks and the baby weighed 3.2 kg (7 lb) – I spent absolutely no time at all in hospital other than going into hospital as I went into labour. Why was there such a big change in treatment?

The last 15 years have seen a dramatic change in our attitudes to the care of pregnancy in women with diabetes. Good blood glucose control is the most important goal and with home blood glucose monitoring this can be achieved in the majority of women without the need for admission to hospital at any stage. It sounds as if your control was worse during your first pregnancy than your second. Early delivery by caesarean section was decided on because the baby had already grown to 3.7 kg by 36 weeks and the doctors were worried that it would become even bigger if left to 38 or 39 weeks. The heavier baby in the first pregnancy was because the high blood glucose you were running resulted in more fat being laid down on the baby. However, during your second pregnancy, when your control was clearly a good deal better, the baby grew at a more normal rate, so that it was at the correct weight when you went into labour at the end of pregnancy.

During my last labour I was given a drip and had an insulin pump up all day. Why was this necessary?

Strict blood glucose control during labour is very important to ensure that you do not put your baby at risk from hypoglycaemia in the first few hours of life. If there is any possibility that your labour may end up with an anaesthetic (e.g. for forceps delivery or possible caesarean section), then the simplest way to keep your diabetes well controlled is with glucose being run into your circulation and matched with an appropriate dose of insulin. With the pump this means that – should an emergency arise – you will be immediately ready.

During my pregnancy I found attending the antenatal clinic a nuisance and I did not like to keep my diabetes too well controlled because, if I did, I had many hypos. Labour and delivery seemed to go quite normally but my baby was rather heavy. He was 4.2 kg (9 lb 4 oz), and had to spend a long time in the Special Care Baby Unit because they said he was hypoglycaemic – how do I avoid all this trouble in my next pregnancy?

If you want to go ahead and have further babies, then it is essential that you change your attitude to the antenatal clinic and to controlling your diabetes throughout the pregnancy. The trouble that your baby had from hypoglycaemia was a reflection of the fact that he had been exposed to a very high glucose concentration throughout pregnancy and had had to produce a lot of insulin from his own pancreas to cope with this extra load of glucose from you. Immediately after birth he no longer had the glucose coming from you but still had too much insulin of his own, hence the hypoglycaemia.

You can prevent this risk in future pregnancies by ensuring that your control is immaculate. This will require you to attend the antenatal clinic on a regular basis and to do frequent blood glucose monitoring to ensure that your control is excellent. If you can do this you should be able to eliminate any risk of hypoglycaemia in your baby.

Is it all right for me to breastfeed my baby if my blood glucose is too high?

Breastfeeding is generally encouraged these days for all women with babies. There are no special difficulties for women with diabetes and the presence of a slightly raised blood glucose need not worry you too much, provided that your control of your diabetes is not too bad. For the best results with breastfeeding, keep up a high fluid intake and keep an eye on your diabetes, making appropriate adjustments to your insulin dose if necessary. Breastfeeding is a demanding process in terms of increasing nutritional requirements for anyone, so make sure that you eat regular amounts of carbohydrate to minimize the risk of hypo-glycaemia. If you find this all too much, it is perfectly all right to bottle-feed. Do not breastfeed whilst having a hypo – feed your-self first, so that you and your baby will both be satisfied! Always seek medical advice if you are in any doubt.

My diabetes was fairly easy to control during my pregnancy, but since the birth of my baby it has been more difficult to control, and I am needing much less insulin. I am breastfeeding – could this have anything to do with it?

Various hormones are produced during pregnancy and these lead to an increase in your insulin requirements and alter your body's metabolism in such a way that obtaining good control is usually easier. After the birth these hormones decrease which means that you need much less insulin, and in many people this dose is even lower than was required before pregnancy. When you are breastfeeding, the dose usually drops even more and you should be prepared to lower your dose of insulin should hypos occur.

I am married to a man who takes insulin to control his diabetes. I have just fallen pregnant, so what special things do I need to do during pregnancy to ensure that it goes smoothly and without complications?

You need take no special precautions other than those taken by all pregnant women, as the fact that your husband has diabetes does not put your pregnancy at any particular risk. It is only when the mother has diabetes that strict control and careful monitoring of blood glucose become essential.

I have been told that I must keep my blood glucose levels as low as possible during pregnancy. Please can you tell me what they should be?

Your blood glucose before meals should be 4–6 mmol/litre and 2 hours after meals no higher than 5–8 mmol/litre.

I am frightened of having hypoglycaemic attacks especially as I have been told to keep my blood glucose much lower during pregnancy. What should I do?

All people treated with insulin should be prepared for a hypo whether or not they are pregnant (there is a section on *Hypos* in Chapter 3). Carry glucose or dextrose or something like a mini-Mars bar on you at all times. Most convenient are Dextro-energy tablets. Some people prefer to carry small (125 ml) cans of Lucozade or Coca-Cola (not the diet variety).

Will any hypoglycaemic attacks that I might have during pregnancy harm the baby?

No. There is no evidence to suggest that even a very low blood glucose in the mother can harm the baby.

Complications

My second son was born with multiple defects and has subsequently died. I have been on insulin for 14 years (since the age of 10). Are women with diabetes more likely to have an abnormal baby?

The secret to a successful pregnancy is perfect blood glucose control starting before conception and continuing throughout pregnancy. There is good scientific evidence to suggest that multiple developmental defects are caused by poor control in the first few weeks of pregnancy and that the risk of this can be avoided by ensuring immaculate control at the time that the baby is conceived. The risks in terms of multiple congenital defects seem to be confined to the very early stages of the pregnancy. This is hardly surprising because this is the stage when the various components of the baby's body are beginning to develop and when other illnesses such as German measles (rubella) also affect development.

Good control is also needed for the rest of the pregnancy because the gradual development and growth of the baby can be disturbed by poor control. In particular, with poor control, the baby grows rather faster than normal and is large in size, although the development of the organs remains relatively immature in terms of their function. This does not happen with well-controlled diabetes. Because the baby is large, the mother has to be delivered early and, because the baby is immature, it is susceptible to a number of added risks immediately after birth.

I have read that the babies of mothers with diabetes tend to be fat and have lung trouble shortly after birth and also there is a risk of hypoglycaemia. Is this true, and if so why does it happen?

We know that, if the mother runs a high blood glucose throughout pregnancy, glucose gets across the placenta into the baby's circulation and causes the baby to become fat. This is because the baby's pancreas is still capable of producing insulin even though the mother's cannot. As a result of this, the baby grows bigger during pregnancy and delivery has to be carried out earlier to avoid a difficult labour. This used to be carried out most commonly by caesarean section at about 36 weeks of pregnancy. One of the complications of this method of delivery is lung trouble in these babies, known as the respiratory distress syndrome (RDS), caused by the fact that the babies were born before their lungs were properly developed.

If the mother's blood glucose levels are kept strictly within normal limits during pregnancy, babies do not grow faster than they should and pregnancy can be allowed to continue for the normal period of 40 weeks. This avoids the risk of caesarean section in the majority of women and RDS is rarely seen because the babies are fully mature when they are born.

Low blood glucose (hypoglycaemia) during the first few hours after birth is a result of the fact that the baby's pancreas has been producing a lot of insulin during the pregnancy to cover the mother's high blood glucose, which was passed across the placenta to the baby. If the mother's blood glucose is strictly controlled during pregnancy and delivery, hypoglycaemia in the baby is much less of a problem.

My baby was born with jaundice. Are babies of mothers with diabetes more likely to have this?

Babies born to mothers with diabetes are more likely to be jaundiced. This is partly because they tend to be born early, but we do not know why a mature baby is jaundiced, though the problem is usually mild and clears without treatment.

I developed toxaemia during my last pregnancy and had to spend several weeks in hospital even though control of my diabetes was immaculate. Luckily everything turned out all right and I now have a beautiful healthy son. Was the toxaemia related to me having diabetes? Is it likely to recur in future pregnancies?

Women with diabetes are more prone to toxaemia. You are not more likely to develop toxaemia in your future pregnancies – indeed the risk is less.

During my last pregnancy I had 'hydramnios' and my obstetrician said that this was because I had diabetes. Is this true? And is there anything that I can do to avoid it happening in future pregnancies?

Hydramnios is an excessive amount of fluid surrounding the fetus and it is, unfortunately, more common in mothers with diabetes. It does appear to be related to how strictly you control your diabetes throughout your pregnancy. Our advice is that you can reduce the risk to an absolute minimum in future pregnancies by aiming to keep your HbA_{1c} and blood glucose levels completely normal from the day of conception.

During the recent delivery of my fourth child (which went quite smoothly) I had an insulin pump into a vein during labour. I had not had this in my previous three pregnancies, despite having diabetes. Why did I need the pump this time?

We now know that it is very important to keep your blood glucose within normal limits during labour to minimize the risk of your baby developing a low blood glucose (hypoglycaemia) in the first few hours after birth. This is most effectively and easily done using an intravenous insulin infusion combined with some glucose given as an intravenous drip. This means that your blood glucose can be kept strictly regulated at the normal level until your baby has been delivered. It also ensures that should any complications arise and something like a caesarean section be required, you are all ready immediately for an anaesthetic and operation.

My first child was delivered by caesarean section. Do I have to have a caesarean section with my next pregnancy?

It all depends on why you had the caesarean section. If it was performed for an obstetric reason that is likely to be present in this pregnancy, then the answer is yes. If it was performed because the first baby was large or just because you have diabetes, the answer could be no.

Some doctors do consider it safer to deliver a woman by caesarean section if she has had a caesarean section before. Others would allow you a 'trial of labour'. In other words, you would start labour and, if everything was satisfactory, you would be able to deliver your baby vaginally in the normal way.

My doctor tells me that I will have to have a caesarean section because my baby is in a bad position and a little large. What sort of anaesthetic is best?

Nowadays approximately 50% of women who have caesarean sections have them under epidural anaesthetic rather than under general anaesthetic. If you have an epidural anaesthetic your legs and abdomen are made completely numb by injecting local anaesthetic solution through a needle into the epidural space in your spine. You remain awake for the birth of your baby and therefore remember this event. In most cases an epidural is preferred because your baby receives none of the anaesthetic and therefore is not sleepy.

If you are interested in having your baby this way, you should discuss it with your obstetrician.

My baby had difficulty with breathing in his first few days in the Special Care Unit. They said this was because my control of my diabetes was poor – why was this?

It sounds as if your baby had what is called respiratory distress syndrome (RDS) which occurs most commonly in premature babies and was discussed in an earlier question. It occurs in babies of mothers with diabetes where the baby has grown too quickly because of the mother's poor blood glucose control, and so the baby is born before it has become fully mature. It used to be a relatively common cause of death in the babies of mothers with diabetes but now, because of stricter control and supervision, the mother does not have to be delivered early, so the baby is fully mature when it is born. It is now uncommon and indeed you can probably completely prevent it if you control your blood glucose throughout your pregnancy, thus allowing it to proceed for the normal 40 weeks.

8
Diabetes in the young

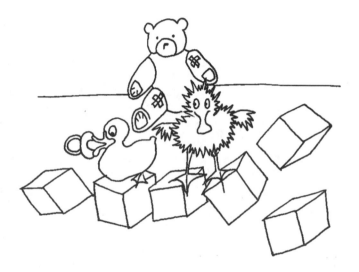

This chapter about diabetes in young people divides naturally into three main age groups: babies, children and adolescents. The sections on babies and children consist of questions asked by parents and the answers are naturally directed at them. The section on adolescents is for both young people and their parents.

Apart from the experience of Diabetes UK camps, none of the authors has actually lived with the daily problems of bringing up a child with diabetes. However, we have listened to hundreds of parents who have felt the despair of finding that their child has diabetes and then overcome their fears to allow their child to develop to the full. Mothers and fathers usually end up by being especially proud of children who have diabetes. We hope to pass on some of this experience to those parents who are still at the frightened stage.

The baby with diabetes

My baby developed diabetes when she was 4 weeks old. She is now 6 weeks old and looks very healthy but I would like emergency advice in order to protect her life. What food and treatment should I give her?

You must be relieved that your baby is better now that she has started treatment, but worried about the difficulties of bringing up a child with diabetes from infancy. Diabetes is very rare in infants less than 12 months old, so you will not find many doctors with experience of this condition. However, the general principles are the same for all infants with diabetes and there is no reason why she should not grow into a healthy young woman.

Diabetes UK has produced a special youth pack for children under 5 years old, which contains many useful documents including a booklet about babies with diabetes. Diabetes UK might also be able to put you in touch with other people who have had the same problem. Practical advice and reassurance from these people would be more use than any theoretical advice.

Like all babies, your daughter will be fed on breast or bottle milk. For the first 4 months frequent feeds are best – 3-hourly by day and 4-hourly by night. Bottle-fed babies usually need 1 scoop (168 g of milk per kg of body weight) each day (2½ ounces per pound). Some babies grow very rapidly and need more milk than this, while others may need solids earlier than 4 months. This may be a help in babies with diabetes as the solids will slow down the absorption of milk. It is important to wake young babies for a night feed to avoid night-time insulin reactions. If there is any doubt about this, do a blood glucose check while your baby is asleep. If her blood glucose is low an additional 5–10 g carbohydrate (100–200 ml milk) should be given.

My little boy is nearly 12 months old and has been ill for a month, losing weight and always crying. Diabetes has just been diagnosed. Does this mean injections for life?

Yes. We are afraid it does literally mean injections for life. The thought of having to stick needles into a young child quite naturally horrifies parents, but with loving care, explanations and playing games like injecting yourself (without insulin) and a teddy bear (using a different needle) and perhaps some bribery, most children accept injections as part of their normal day. Young children grow up knowing no other way of life and they often accept this treatment better than their parents do. Encourage your child to help at injection time by getting the equipment ready or perhaps by pushing in the plunger and pulling out the needle.

How can I collect urine for testing from my 18-month-old son? I have been given lots of different suggestions but none of them seems to work.

It is not easy to get clean samples of urine from babies in nappies. Many infants will produce a specimen by reflex into a small potty when undressed. You can also squeeze a wet nappy directly onto a urine testing stick. But be warned – washing powders or fabric softeners in the nappies alter the urine test result.

Diastix or Diabur-Test 5000 can be used for testing for glucose, whilst Ketostix or Ketur Test are used to test for ketones. Keto-Diastix and Keto-Diabur tests for glucose and ketones. Infants are much more likely than older people to have ketones in the urine. This is because they rapidly switch to burning up fat stores in the fasting state. It is important to check on ketones and try to keep his urine ketone-free, although you should not worry if ketones appear for a short time.

You will also have to do blood tests on your son. Parents expect children to find these painful but blood tests taken from a finger, heel or ear lobe are surprisingly well accepted by young people. They enable you to check accurately what is happening if your son feels unwell or looks ill. Urine tests provide only a guide about the state of his diabetes since his last urine specimen. The blood test confirms what is happening at that very instant. It is the only reliable way of deciding whether your son is hypo or just tired and hungry. Blood glucose measurements are also necessary to check the overall control of his diabetes and to help you decide on the dose of insulin if his blood glucose rises during an illness. Blood samples should be obtained with an automatic finger pricker – the Autolet (Owen Mumford [Medical Shop]) has a special platform for children, but the Soft Touch and Softclix (Roche), the Glucolet (Bayer Diagnostics), the BD Lancer (BD) and the Monojector (Tyco Healthcare) are all suitable. Addresses for all these suppliers are given in Appendix 3. There are new blood glucose meters on the market that need only a very small amount of blood for the test. For instance, the OneTouch Ultra works on a tiny blood sample and comes with a new lancing device, which is adjustable. The small blood volume means that only the shallowest skin puncture is needed. Adults can check their glucose by sampling from their arm and it is virtually painless. Such a meter would be ideal for a baby or young child.

My 2-year-old daughter has diabetes and makes an awful fuss about food. Meals are turning into a regular struggle. Have you any suggestions?

Food is of great emotional significance to all children. If meals are eaten without complaint, then both mother and child will be satisfied. All children go through phases of food refusal because of a need to show their growing independence, their ability to provoke worry or anger in parents and their attempts to manipulate the situation. Food leads to the well-known battleground, which occurs in all families at some stage. The only way for you to win is to remain in control of the weapon. Usually when young children begin this phase (at 10–18 months), they dislike being told to leave the table and go away. They often return and eat rather than remain alone and hungry.

The battle is even more difficult for parents like you where the child has diabetes – your daughter has some explosive weapons! However, you must stay in control: try distracting her attention away from food by toys, music, talk or your own relaxed

FOOD AND YOUR CHILDREN

Dos and don'ts for babies and toddlers

- Do introduce your baby and toddler to the mashed-up version of the foods and tastes you relish, including the herbs and spices.
- Do clip a baby seat on to the table if possible so that the baby can be part of family eating and have her interest in what you are eating stimulated.
- Do respect your baby or toddler when they say 'no'. When they turn away from eating, offer them some other food and if it doesn't hit the spot, allow them to stop eating. They will soon let you know if they are hungry again.
- Do let your baby and toddler muck about with food and make a mess. Food is a source of creativity as well as fuel.
- Don't encourage them to eat five more spoonfuls for grandma, or the starving children elsewhere, or play games that trick them into eating. Show them your relish in food.

Dos and don'ts for primary-age children

- Do put lots of different kinds of food out and let the children choose what they fancy.
- Don't differentiate between kids' and adult food. Children's tastes will be as complex and sophisticated as the foods they are exposed to.
- Do value foods equally so that broccoli becomes no less of a special food than ice cream.
- Do let children see you stopping when you are full and leaving food on your plate.
- Do let children leave food when they've had enough or when they are compelled to rush off to do something more interesting than eat. If you are worried they have not had enough to eat, make sure there is food around for them to come back and refuel on.
- Don't ever reward them for eating their greens by offering them sweets or ice cream or cake. Do let them eat in whatever order they like including having dessert first if they are desperate for the carbohydrates.
- Don't cheer them up or jolly them out of a sad or angry mood with food unless you know they are hungry. Do let them tell you how they feel without shushing them or humouring them out of their upset. If they tell you and get their feelings out in the open, the pain will dissipate faster.

FOOD AND YOUR CHILDREN (cont'd)

Dos and don'ts for adolescents

- Do expect them to eat fast food. It's a sign of independence, of showing how different they are from you, of making it with their peers. If you've fed them interesting food all along, don't despair, they won't be able to eat KFC or Wagamama every day.
- Do sit together around the table several nights a week. If they've stocked up on food after school and aren't hungry, let them sit with you while you eat so that they get accustomed to being around food and only eating it when they are hungry.
- Don't have fights while eating together. It fuses food and conflict together.
- Do have tons of food in the house and expect erratic eating. Teenagers have fast metabolisms and many need to eat lots more than adults.
- Do tolerate their cooking even if their experiments violate your basic principles in the kitchen.
- Do discourage them from dieting. Set the example by never doing it yourself.
- Don't have a corner for 'junk' food. Disperse it among the foods you consider good.

---

approach to eating. You may have to send your daughter away from the table if she is refusing to eat properly. Hypoglycaemia often provokes hunger and, anyway, a couple of mild hypos due to food refusal are a small price to pay for better behaviour next time. Be prepared to modify the type of carbohydrate within reason if she consistently refuses the diet recommended by the hospital. Bread, potatoes, biscuits, fruit juices and even ice cream can be offered as alternatives.

Susie Orbach has recently written an excellent book called *On eating*. The box reprints the advice that was given in *The Guardian* (reproduced with permission from AP Watt Ltd on behalf of Susie Orbach).

The child with diabetes

My 5-year-old son has had diabetes since he was 18 months and he is only 3' 2" (96 cm) tall. I have been told that he is very short for his age. The doctor says that poorly controlled diabetes could be slowing his growth. Is this true?

The average height for a 5-year -old boy is 3' 6" (108 cm), so your son is certainly short for his age. Having high glucose levels for several years could be the cause of this. If you now keep his diabetes under control and make sure that he has plenty to eat, he should grow rapidly and may even catch up with his normal height. However, his short stature may be due to a growth disorder and may need further investigation.

I have been told not to expect my daughter to be as tall as she would have been had she not had diabetes. Is this true? If so, what can I do to help her reach her maximum height?

Unless your daughter's diabetes control has been very poor, there is no reason why she should not reach her proper height without any special encouragement. We know of one 16-year-old boy who is 6' 2" (165.8 cm) tall and has had diabetes for 15 years. Diabetes does not have to stunt your growth.

My 6-year-old daughter has had diabetes for 4 years. She is on 12 units of Monotard insulin, once a day. Her urine test in the morning is always 2% and the teatime test 1%. My own doctor is satisfied with her tests and says that negative tests in a child of this age mean a risk of hypos. However, the school doctor says her diabetes is out of control and she should have two injections a day. What do you advise?

Until a few years ago most doctors did not try to achieve close control of diabetes in children. It was considered good enough if the child felt well and was not having a lot of hypos. The feeling nowadays is that good control is important to allow normal growth and prevent long-term complications.

In the first place, you should start measuring your daughter's blood glucose. This will tell you how serious her early morning high glucose actually is, and also whether she is running the risk of a hypo at any other time of the day. It is likely that she will need an evening injection to control her morning blood glucose.

It is true that keeping her blood glucose down towards normal may make a hypo more likely. Mild hypos do not cause any harm and even severe reactions do no damage, except to the parent's confidence! You must not worry about a few days or weeks of poor control and you will never achieve perfection in a little girl whose activities and lifestyle are changing daily.

My son, aged 10, started insulin last year and his dose has gradually dropped. Now he has come off insulin completely and is on diet alone. Will he now be off insulin permanently?

No. There is a 99.9% chance that he will have to go back on insulin. This so-called 'honeymoon period' (there is more about this in the section on *Insulin* in Chapter 3) can be very trying as it raises hopes that the diabetes has cleared up. Unfortunately, this very, very rarely happens in young people.

Are there any special schools for children with diabetes?

There are no special schools for children with diabetes and they would not be a good idea. It is most important that young people with diabetes grow up in normal surroundings and are not encouraged to regard themselves as 'different'. These children should go to normal schools and grow up in a normal family atmosphere.

I think my newly diagnosed son is using his insulin injections as a way of avoiding school. I can't send him to school unless he has his insulin but it sometimes takes ages before I can get him to have his injection. I have two younger children and a husband whom I also have to help to get to school and work. How should I cope with my temperamental son?

You raise several related points. Firstly, you assume that he is using his insulin injections to avoid school. You may be right if he resisted going to school before developing diabetes. In this case you should try the same tactics that you used before. Alternatively, his dislike of school could be related to the diabetes, for example an overprotective attitude by sports instructors, frequent hypos or embarrassment about eating snacks between meals. If you suspect such difficulties, a talk to your son and his form teacher might clear the air.

He may in fact be happy about school but actually frightened of his insulin injections so that things get off to a slow start in the morning. Problems with injections have been reduced with the introduction of insulin pens, but some children focus their dislike for diabetes as a whole on the unnatural process of injecting themselves.

Diabetes UK has produced an Information for Schools and Youth Organizations Pack to help parents communicate with the school. It contains information to be given to teachers and those responsible for children with diabetes. You can contact Diabetes UK (the address is in Appendix 3) for a copy of this publication.

When my son starts school, would it be better for him to return home for lunch or let him eat school dinners?

It depends largely on your son's temperament and attitude to school. Some 4-year-olds skip happily off to their first day at school without a backward glance (much to their mother's chagrin), while other perfectly normal children make a fuss and have tummy aches at the start of school. Diabetes will tend to add to these problems. You will have to talk to his teachers and it would be worth asking their advice and making sure that someone will take the responsibility of choosing suitable food for your son – you can't leave that to a 4- or 5-year-old child.

My 10-year-old son has recently been diagnosed with diabetes. What is the best age for him to start doing his own injections?

The fear of injections may loom large in a child's view of his own diabetes. Many children actually make less fuss if they do their own injections and most diabetes specialist nurses would encourage a 10-year-old to do his own injections right from day one. We know a girl who developed diabetes at the age of 6 and who gave herself her own first injection without any fuss – and has been doing so ever since. Insulin pens take a lot of the horror out of injections.

If you do have an injection problem or if you want your son to have a good summer holiday, encourage him to go on a Diabetes UK holiday – you will find details in *Balance* or contact the care interventions team of Diabetes UK (address in Appendix 3).

When I heard that I was to have a child with diabetes in my class (I am a junior school teacher), I read up all I could about diabetes. Most of my questions were answered but I cannot discover what to do if the child eats too much sugar. Will he go into a coma? If so, what do I do then?

Eating sugar or sweets may make his blood glucose rise in which case he may feel thirsty and generally off-colour. Coma from a high blood glucose takes some time to develop and there is only cause for concern if he becomes very drowsy or starts vomiting. If this does happen, you should contact his parents. A child who is vomiting with poor diabetes control probably needs to go to hospital.

The most common sort of coma, which may occur over a matter of 10 minutes, is due to a hypo. In this case the blood glucose level is too low and he needs to be given sugar at once.

The causes of hypo are delayed meals, missed snacks or extra exercise.

Can I apply for an allowance to look after my son who has frequent hypos and needs a lot of extra care?

Yes, as the parent of a child with unstable diabetes you can apply for a disability living allowance, which is a non-means-tested benefit. Many people in your position have successfully applied and feel that it provides some recognition of the burden of being responsible for a child with diabetes, especially if hypos are a major problem. There is more information about Social Security benefits in Chapter 5.

There is an opposing view that diabetes should not be regarded as a disability and that applying for an allowance fosters a feeling that the child is an invalid.

My little boy has diabetes and is always having coughs and colds. These make him very ill and he always becomes very sugary during each illness despite antibiotics from my doctor. Could you please give me some guidelines for coping with his diabetes during these infections?

Yes, of course. The main guidelines are shown in the box on the facing page.

I am headmaster of a school for deaf children and one of my pupils developed diabetes two years ago. Since then his learning ability has deteriorated and I wondered if this had any connection with his diabetes?

No. Diabetes in itself has no effect on learning ability and there are plenty of children with diabetes who excel academically. Poorly controlled diabetes with a very high blood glucose could reduce his powers of concentration. Hypoglycaemic attacks are usually short lasting but he could be missing a few key items while his blood glucose is low and be unable to catch up.

At a psychological level, the double handicap of deafness and

COPING WITH DIABETES DURING INFECTIONS

Insulin

- Never stop the insulin even if your son is vomiting. During feverish illnesses the body often needs more insulin, not less.
- During an illness it may be useful to use only clear (short-acting) insulin.
- You may have to give three or four injections a day as this is much more flexible and so you can respond more quickly to changes in the situation.
- Give one-third of the total daily insulin dose in the morning, as clear insulin only.

Food

- Stop solid food but give him sugary drinks, e.g. Lucozade 60 ml (10 g) or orange squash with two teaspoons of sugar (10 g).
- Milk drinks and yoghurt are an acceptable alternative for ill children.
- Aim to give 10–20 g of carbohydrate every hour.

Blood tests

- At midday, check his blood glucose and, if it is 13 mmol/litre or more, give the same dose of clear insulin as in the morning plus an extra 2 units.
- Repeat this process every 4–6 hours, increasing the dose of insulin if the blood glucose remains high.
- Once he is better, cut the insulin back to the original dose.

Ketones

- Check his urine for ketones twice daily. If these are +++, either your son needs more food or his diabetes is going badly out of control.

Vomiting

- Young children who vomit more than two or three times should always be seen by a doctor or specialist nurse to help supervise the illness. They can become dehydrated in the space of a few hours and if vomiting continues they will need fluid dripped into a vein. Unfortunately this means a hospital admission.

diabetes could be affecting his morale and self-confidence. Perhaps he would be helped by meeting other boys of his age who also have diabetes. This often helps children to realize that diabetes is compatible with normal life and activities. Contact Diabetes UK who can help you in this area.

My son was recently awarded a scholarship to a well-known public school but when they found he had diabetes, he was refused admission on medical grounds. They can give no positive reason for this and our consultant has tried very hard to make them change their minds. Why should he be so penalized?

This was a disgraceful decision based on old-fashioned prejudice. It looks as if nothing will make the school change its mind but, if Diabetes UK were told, they might have brought more pressure to bear. The Disability Discrimination Act will also cover access to education. You could also consider seeking legal advice.

Should my son tell his school friends about his diabetes?

It is very important that your son tells his close friends that he has diabetes. He should explain about hypos and tell them that, if he does behave in an odd way, they should make him take sugar and he should show them where he keeps his supplies. If your son shows his friends how he measures his blood glucose, they will almost certainly be interested in diabetes and be keen to help him with it. We know several young people who bring their closest friend to the hospital diabetes clinic with them. As he becomes older and spends more time away from home, your son will come to depend more on his friends.

**My 10-year-old son moves on to a large comprehensive
school in a few months time. Up until now he has been
in a small junior school where all the staff know about
his diabetes. I worry that he will be swamped in the
'big' school where he will come across lots of different
teachers who know nothing about his condition. Have
you any advice on this problem?**

Moving up to a big comprehensive school is always a daunting
experience and is bound to cause the parents of a child with diabetes extra worry. The important thing is to go and talk to your
son's form teacher, preferably before the first day of term when
he or she will have hundreds of new problems to cope with.
Assume that the teacher knows nothing about diabetes and try to
get across the following points.

- Make sure that they know your child needs daily insulin
  injections.
- He may need to eat at certain unusual times.
- Describe how your son behaves when hypo and emphasize
  the importance of giving him sugar. If he is hypo do not
  send him to the school office or to home alone.
- Staggered lunch hours may be a problem as he may need to
  eat at a fixed time each day.
- If he needs a lunchtime injection, then you need to arrange
  with his teachers how he should store and have access to
  his insulin, syringe or insulin pen, and blood testing
  equipment.
- You will need to be told if he is going to be kept in late (e.g.
  for detention) as parents tend to worry if their children fail
  to show up.
- Ask the form teacher to make sure all your son's other
  teachers know these facts.

Diabetes UK supplies a School Pack, which should help explain
diabetes to his teachers and it is especially important to speak
personally to his sports and swimming instructors. If there are
problems with the school over such things as sports, outings or
school meals, your diabetes clinic may have a diabetes specialist

nurse or health visitor who could go to the school and explain things. You will probably have to repeat this exercise at the beginning of every school year.

What arrangements can I make with school about my 9-year-old daughter's special requirements for school dinners?

It is important to go and see the head teacher and preferably the caterer to explain that your daughter must have her dinner on time. Explain that she needs a certain amount of carbohydrate in a form that she will eat and that she should avoid puddings containing sugar. If your diabetes clinic has a diabetes specialist nurse or health visitor, she may be able to go to the school and give advice.

Most parents of children with diabetes get round the whole problem by providing a packed lunch. This means that you have more control over what your daughter eats and you can supply the sort of food she likes and what is good for her. Point out to your daughter that it would be best for her to eat the contents of her own lunch box, and not to swap them with other children!

When she goes on to secondary school she may be faced with a cafeteria system. This should allow her to choose suitable food but she may also choose unsuitable items and try to exist on jam doughnuts.

My son has diabetes. Can I allow him to go on school trips?

In general the answer is yes, but for your own peace of mind you would want to be satisfied that one of the staff on the trip would be prepared to take responsibility for your son. Day trips should be no problem as long as someone can be sure that he eats on time and has his second injection if necessary. At junior school level, long trips away from home, especially on the continent, could be more difficult and it really depends on you finding a member of staff that you can trust. They will need to keep an eye on your son and to know how to cope sensibly with problems like a bad hypo. Once in secondary school most children manage to go away on trips with the school, scouts or a youth group. Of course one of the adults in the party should be responsible, but as your son gets older he will be better able to look after himself. Diabetes UK has the following check list for things to take on school trips and holidays:

- identification necklace or bracelet
- glucose
- insulin, insulin pen (or syringe), needles
- testing equipment for blood glucose
- food to cover journeys with extra for unexpected delays
- Hypostop Gel.

This is part of the Information for Schools and Youth Organizations Pack, which is available from Diabetes UK – the address is in Appendix 3.

My 10-year-old child has heard about Diabetes UK camps from the clinic. I am a bit worried about letting him go off on his own for two weeks. Do you not think that I should wait a few years before sending him to a camp?

No, he's not too young to go. Diabetes UK has been organizing holidays for children since the 1930s and it has become an enormous enterprise. About 500 children take part in these holidays each year, so in one sense your son will not be on his own. Young children love going on group holidays, and the fact of being with other children with diabetes gives them a great sense of confidence – for once they are not the odd ones out. The children learn a great deal from each other and from the staff. Your son will have an exciting holiday and you will have a few weeks off from worrying about his diabetes.

Is it safe to let my little girl go on a Diabetes UK camp?

Perfectly safe. The care interventions team of Diabetes UK has had years of experience in running holidays for children. The average camp consists of 30–35 children who are supervised by the following staff:

- Warden, responsible for planning
- Senior Medical Officer, who is experienced in diabetes
- Junior Medical Officer
- 2–4 Nurses, usually with a special interest in diabetes and/or children
- 3 Dietitians
- 1–2 Deputy Wardens
- 8 Junior Leaders, young adults with diabetes themselves, who give up two weeks to help.

The staff/child ratio is about 1:2 and there is always close supervision on outings and all sports, especially swimming.

Diabetes and the adolescent

My 16-year-old son is only 5' 2" (157 cm) and very immature. I have heard that children with diabetes reach puberty a year or two later than anyone else. Will he grow later?

If your son is sexually underdeveloped, then he will certainly have a growth spurt when he goes into puberty. However, 5' 2" (157 cm) is undersized for a boy of 16. It could be poor diabetes control that has stunted his growth but there are other possible factors, including the physical stature of his father and yourself. If you are both a normal height, there could be some other medical reason for your son's short size. It would be worth consulting your GP or clinic doctor rather than blaming it automatically on his diabetes.

My daughter and I are getting extremely anxious although our GP tells us there is nothing to worry about. She developed diabetes when she was 14 years old, 1 year after her periods had started. They stopped completely with the diabetes and have never started again, although we have now waited for 2 years. Is our GP right to be calm and patient, or are we right to be worried?

A major upset to the system such as diabetes may cause periods to stop in a young girl. It is a little unusual for them not to reappear within 2 years and we should like to be certain that your daughter's diabetes is well controlled and that she is not underweight. Your doctor will be able to answer these two questions. If her control is good and she is of normal weight, then it would be reasonable to wait 1 or 2 years before embarking on further investigations. There is a very good chance that her periods will return spontaneously. If they do not return, nothing will be lost by waiting for another 2 years.

I am nearly 16 and have not started menstruating yet. Is this because I have diabetes? Since I was diagnosed, I have put on a lot of weight.

On average, girls with diabetes do tend to start their periods at an older age. We assume from your question that you are now overweight and this may be another cause for delay in menstruation. Presumably you have begun to notice other signs of puberty such as breast development and the growth of pubic hair. If so, you should make a determined effort to lose weight and control your diabetes carefully. This will involve a reduction in your food intake and probably an adjustment in your dose of insulin. If, after another year, you have still not seen a period then you should discuss the matter with your doctor.

My son has just heard that he will be going to university next year. While we are all delighted and proud of him, I worry because he will be living away from home for the first time. For the 7 years since he was diagnosed, I have accepted most of the anxiety and practical arrangement of his meals and he has done his best to ignore his diabetes. How is he now going to face it alone?

If your son is bright enough to get into university, he should be quite capable of looking after his diabetes. However, you are right to point out that your son's attitude towards his diabetes is also important. All mothers worry when their children leave home for the first time and it is natural for a child with diabetes to cause extra worry. You can be sure, however, that the training you have given him over the years will bear fruit. Most children like to spread their wings when first leaving home and you can expect a period of adjustment to his new responsibilities. Provided that he realizes why you regard good control of his diabetes as important, he will probably become more responsible in good time. It would also be sensible for your son to contact the diabetes clinic in his university town, so that they can give him support if necessary.

How does diabetes affect my prospects for marriage?

We have never heard a young man or woman complain that diabetes has put off potential marriage partners, although we suppose it could be used as an excuse if someone was looking for a convenient way out of a relationship.

If your diabetes has affected your own self-confidence and made you feel a second-class citizen, then you may sell yourself short and lose out in that way.

I have Type 1 diabetes and have recently made friends with a super boy but am frightened that he will be put off if I tell him I have diabetes. What should I do?

The standard answer is that you must tell your new boyfriend at the beginning. However, you have obviously found this a problem or you would not be asking the question. There is no need to broadcast the fact that you have diabetes. It would be possible to conceal diabetes completely from a close companion, although sooner or later he will inevitably discover the truth.

Once you get to know him better, your best plan would be to drop a few hints about diabetes without making a song and dance about it, perhaps during a meal together. If the relationship grows, you will want to share each other's problems – including diabetes. We have never known a serious relationship break up because of diabetes.

My 15-year-old son developed diabetes at the age of 12. Initially he was very sensible about his diabetes but recently he has become resentful saying that he is different from everyone else and blaming us for his disease. What do you suggest?

You must first realize that most people of all ages (and their parents) feel resentful at some stage about this condition, which causes so much inconvenience in someone's life. Many 12-year-old children conform with their parent's wishes and generally do as they are told. However, by the age of 15 other important pressures are beginning to bear on a developing young person. In the case of a boy, the most important factors in life are first his friends and secondly girls – or possibly the other way round! While you as parents are prepared to make allowances and provide special meals for example, most young lads want to join the gang and do not wish to appear 'different'.

At a diabetes camp (which was restricted to hand-picked, well adjusted young adults with diabetes), the organizers were horrified to discover how angry the young people felt about their condition. Of course this anger will often be directed at the parents. We can only give advice in general terms that apply to most adolescent problems.

- Keep lines of communication open.
- Boost his self-esteem by giving praise where praise is due even if your own self-esteem is taking a hammering.

- Allow your son to make his own decisions about diabetes. If you force him to comply, he will simply avoid confrontation by deceiving you.
- Remember that difficult adolescents usually turn into successful adults.

Our 15-year-old daughter has had diabetes for 4 years and until recently has always been well controlled. Now it is very difficult to get her to take an interest in her diabetes and she has stopped doing blood tests. At the last clinic visit, the doctor said that her HbA$_{1c}$ was very high and he thought she was probably missing some of her injections. I really do not know what to do.

This is a very upsetting situation for all concerned and unfortunately it is not uncommon. Diabetes is difficult because it places great demands and restrictions on people but in the short term they have nothing to show for their efforts. Non-compliance (not following the prescribed treatment) is very common and the reasons for it are very complex. Like most girls of her age, your daughter probably wants to lose weight and she may have discovered that allowing her glucose levels to float up is a very effective way of quickly losing a few pounds in weight. Thus there may be positive gain to your daughter in missing a few insulin injections.

There is no easy solution to this problem especially as many girls in this situation brightly turn up at the clinic and announce that 'everything is fine'. Simply challenging your daughter and threatening her with the long-term complications of diabetes is unlikely to do much good. It is better to try and get her to realize that you understand that living with diabetes is not easy, and allow her to express her own feelings about it. Of course she may be at a stage of feeling that parents are light-years away from her own experience in which case she is more likely to unburden herself to a close friend, especially someone else with diabetes.

9

Long-term complications

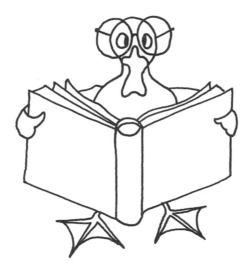

Before insulin was discovered, people with diabetes did not survive long enough to develop diabetic complications as we know them today. In the early days after the great discovery, it was widely believed that insulin cured diabetes. We are now in a better position to realize that, although insulin produced nothing short of miraculous recovery in those on the verge of death and returned them to a full and active life, it is no cure for the condition. However, used properly, insulin results in full health and activity and a long life.

Life expectancy has increased progressively since insulin was first used in 1922 and there are now many thousands of people who have successfully completed more than 50 years of insulin treatment. Increased longevity has brought with it a number of the so-called 'long-term complications', some of which (such as heart disease and gangrene of the legs) occur not uncommonly in people who do not have diabetes and are generally considered to be inevitable consequences of the ageing process (we all have to die some time!). Others are not seen in people without diabetes. These conditions are therefore considered the long-term complications specific to diabetes: the three most important are eye damage (*retinopathy*), nerve damage (*neuropathy*) and kidney damage (*nephropathy*).

Diabetic retinopathy can lead to loss of vision and indeed is the commonest cause of blindness registration in people under 65 in the UK. Fortunately it leads to visual loss only in a small proportion of people. Diabetic neuropathy, by leading to loss of feeling, particularly in the feet, makes affected people susceptible to infections and occasionally gangrene, leading to the risk of amputation. It can also cause impotence. Diabetic nephropathy can cause kidney failure and is now the commonest reason for referral for renal dialysis and transplantation in the UK and Europe in young people, although again it occurs only in very small numbers.

It is not surprising that people dread the thought of diabetic complications. In the past they worried but did not ask about them as they were a taboo subject. They were only for discussion between doctors and not between doctor and patient.

The world has changed and today people rightly demand to know more about their condition ('Whose life is it anyway?') and the majority now find out about the dreaded 'complications' soon after they are diagnosed. There are so many old wives' tales circulating about diabetic complications and it is perhaps the most important area in diabetic counselling where the facts rather than opinions must be stated.

Although medical science has made impressive progress since the discovery of insulin, there is still a long way to go. The scientific evidence from studies of experimental diabetes in animals is strongly in favour of the specific complications of diabetes being directly related to the degree to which the blood glucose is raised. Conversely their prevention is possible by tight control of the blood glucose concentration. We believe that the specific diabetic complications in humans are also a direct result of a raised blood glucose level over many years and that they are all preventable by keeping blood glucose values and HbA_{1c} values normal. This view has been supported by the results of a very large multicentre clinical trial in the USA – the Diabetes Control and Complications Trial (DCCT), and the UK Prospective Diabetes Study (UKPDS) in the UK, which conclusively proved that complications can be avoided by strict blood glucose control. There is more information about the trials in the section on *Control and monitoring* in Chapter 4.

Some of the questions in this chapter relating to eyes and feet are not strictly questions about complications, but as they do not easily fit in anywhere else in the book they have been included in this chapter under their specific headings.

General questions

Can someone who is controlled only by diet suffer from diabetic complications?

Complications may occur with any type of diabetes. The cause of diabetic complications is not completely understood, although bad control of diabetes is the most important predisposing factor. The duration of diabetes (the length of time for which you have had it, diagnosed or not) is also important – complications are rare in the first few years and occur more commonly after many years.

People treated with diet alone are usually diagnosed in middle or later life. At the time of diagnosis, the disease may have been present for a long time, often many years, without the person being aware of it, and therefore without any attempt being made to control it. Thus it is not surprising that complications can occur in some people even when they are treated with diet alone. Good control in these people is clearly just as important as in people who have treatment with tablets or who have Type 1 diabetes.

My child has had diabetes for 3 years and I am trying to find out more about the disease. I recently read a book, which said that some people with diabetes may go blind. I don't know if this is true and find it very upsetting. Surely they shouldn't be allowed to write such things in books that young people might read?

You raise a very important matter. Diabetes was almost always fatal within 1 or 2 years of diagnosis until the outlook was revolutionized by the discovery of insulin. None the less, it still required a lot of work and experimental development in the manufacture of insulin before someone with diabetes was able to lead an almost normal life, with the aid of insulin injections, as they do today.

After several years it became obvious to doctors that some people were developing what we now call 'chronic complications' or 'long-term complications'. It was clear that these took many years to develop. This became the object of a massive research drive, requiring the investment of much effort and many years of work by doctors and other scientists. We now understand how some of these complications occur, and we know how to treat them if they occur. We realize that strict control of diabetes is important in their prevention. For this reason, all doctors and other medical personnel treating people with diabetes spend much of their time and effort trying to help them improve their control and keep their blood glucose as near normal as possible. These complications do not occur in all people by any means, although nowadays, with people living longer than ever before, the complications are becoming more important.

You ask whether facts like these should be made available to people with diabetes. The majority of people like to be correctly informed about their condition, its management and its complications. Modern treatment involves increasing frankness between doctors and patients in discussing all aspects of the condition. A survey among our own patients with diabetes showed the majority expected to be told the facts about complications.

What are the complications and what should I keep a lookout for to ensure that they are picked up as soon as possible?

The complications specific to diabetes are known as diabetic retinopathy, neuropathy and nephropathy. Retinopathy means damage to the retina at the back of the eye. Neuropathy means damage to the nerves. This can affect nerves supplying any part of the body but is generally referred to as either 'peripheral' when affecting nerves supplying muscles and skin, or as 'autonomic' when affecting nerves supplying organs such as the bladder, the bowel and the heart. Nephropathy is damage affecting the kidney, which in the first instance makes them more leaky, so that albumin appears in the urine. At a later stage it may affect the function of the kidneys and in severe cases lead to kidney failure.

The best way of detecting complications early is to visit your doctor or clinic for regular review. Regular attendance at the diabetes clinic is important so that complications can be picked up at an early stage and if necessary treated.

Prevention is, however, clearly better than treatment and, if you can control your diabetes properly, you will be less likely to suffer these complications.

I am very worried that I might develop complications after some years of having diabetes. Is it possible to avoid complications in later life? If so, how?

Yes. We believe that all people could avoid complications if they were able to control their diabetes perfectly from the day that they were diagnosed. There are now many people on record who have gone 50 years or more with Type 1 diabetes and are completely free from any signs of complications.

The best advice we can give you on how to avoid complications is to take the control of your blood glucose and diabetes seriously from the outset and to attend regularly for review and supervision by somebody experienced in the management of people with diabetes. Focus on learning how to look after yourself in such a way that you can achieve and maintain a normal HbA_{1c} level (there is a section on this measurement in Chapter 4). If you can do that and keep your HbA_{1c} normal, you can look forward to a life free from the risk of diabetic complications.

To what extent are the complications of diabetes genetically determined?

This is a very difficult question. Most specialists believe that there is a hereditary factor, which predisposes some people to develop complications and makes others relatively immune from them, but so far scientific proof of this is not very strong.

What is the expected lifespan of someone with Type 1 diabetes and why?

The lifespan depends to a very great extent on how old the person is when the diagnosis is made. The older the person at the time of diagnosis the closer their expected lifespan is to that of someone who does not have diabetes.

Looking back to the past we know that, when diabetes was diagnosed in early childhood, the lifespan of people with Type 1 diabetes was generally reduced, mainly because of premature deaths from heart attacks and kidney failure. We know, however, that the lifespan has improved with better medical care. We believe that the life expectancy of a child diagnosed with diabetes in the 1990s is longer than ever previously possible and may be nearly as good as an equivalent child who does not have diabetes. We also know that longevity is greatest in people who make regular visits to their clinic and who keep their diabetes under strict control. Those who die prematurely are more likely to be those who do not attend clinic regularly, are not being supervised adequately and do not control themselves well, and who smoke. This is why we have kept emphasizing the importance of good control throughout this book.

My diabetes specialist has said that it does not follow that badly controlled people get all the side effects and ill health in later life; often the reverse is true. Is this really so?

There is an element of truth in this but the word 'often' should be replaced by 'very occasionally'. Well controlled people rarely become ill and develop side effects, whereas people who have unstable and unbalanced diabetes often develop ill health and side effects in later life. This has been confirmed by the results of the Diabetes Control and Complications Trial (DCCT) in the USA, and the UK Prospective Study (UKPDS) in the UK – there is more information about these trials in the section on *Control and monitoring* in Chapter 4.

For the last two years my cheeks have become increasingly hollow although my weight is static – is this due to diabetes?

Quite a lot of middle-aged and elderly people become slim up top and pear shaped below, whether or not they have diabetes. However, there is a rare form of diabetes called lipoatrophic diabetes and this could possibly be the explanation for the hollowing of your cheeks. This is not a recognized complication of diabetes but a rare form of the condition. Mention it to your doctor the next time you go to your diabetes clinic.

I have had diabetes for the past 10 years and have recently developed an unsightly skin condition on my shins. I was referred to a skin specialist who told me that it was related to my diabetes and would be very difficult to cure. What is it and why does it occur?

Necrobiosis lipoidica diabeticorum (otherwise known as necrobiosis) is a strange non-infective but unsightly condition that most commonly appears on the shins, although it may occasionally appear elsewhere. It may occur in people years before they develop diabetes or at any time thereafter. Nobody knows much about it and treatment can be very disappointing, but achieving good control of diabetes may help. Local steroid injections and freezing with liquid nitrogen (cryotherapy) have been tried without much success. With time the red raised patches quieten down and usually leave transparent scars. Diabetes UK have a necrobiosis network; this enables people with the condition to get in touch with others. You can contact the Diabetes UK Careline for more information.

Eyes

I had a tendency towards short-sightedness before being diagnosed as having diabetes. Is this likely to increase my chances of developing eye complications later on?

Short-sightedness makes not the slightest difference to developing diabetic eye complications – it has been said that those with severe short-sightedness may actually be less, rather than more, prone to retinopathy.

Vision may vary with changes in diabetes control. Severe changes in blood glucose levels can alter the shape of the lens in the eye and thus alter its focusing capacity. It is therefore common for those people with high blood glucose levels (i.e. with poor control) to have difficulty with distance vision – a situation that changes completely when their diabetes is controlled and their blood glucose reduced. When this occurs, vision changes again, so that a person experiences difficulty with near vision and therefore with reading. This can be very frightening, at least until it is understood. After 2 or 3 weeks, vision always returns to the same state as before diabetes developed.

As someone with diabetes, I know I should have my eyes checked, but how often should this be?

If your diabetes is well controlled and your vision is normal and you have no signs of complications, then once a year is generally sufficient. It is important that you do have your eyes checked once a year by someone trained in this examination, since after many years diabetes can affect the back of the eye (the retina). The routine eye checks are aimed at picking this up at an early stage before it seriously affects your vision and at a stage where it can be effectively treated.

I have just been discovered to have diabetes and the glasses that I have had for several years seem no longer suitable, but my doctor tells me not to get them changed until my diabetes has been brought under control – is this right?

Yes. When the glucose concentration in the body rises, this affects the focusing ability of the eyes, but it is only a temporary effect, and things go back to normal once the glucose has been brought under control. If you change your glasses now you will be able to see better but as soon as your diabetes is brought under control you will need to change them yet again. It is better to follow your doctor's advice and wait until your diabetes has been controlled for at least a month before going to the optician again.

Who is the best person to check my eyes once a year?

This can be done by either the specialist in your diabetes clinic, the specialist in the hospital's eye clinic, your general practitioner or your local ophthalmic optician if they are sufficiently well trained to do this.

You need to undergo two examinations. The first is to test your visual acuity, which is basically your ability to read the letters on the chart down to the correct line. The second is to have the back of your eyes looked at with an ophthalmoscope: this is the more difficult of the two examinations and can be done only by somebody with special training. These days some clinics offer a service to GPs that enables people to have the backs of the eyes photographed: the photographs are then examined by a specialist, and the results are sent to the GP.

Last time I was having my eyes checked from the chart, the nurse made me look through a small pinhole. Why was this?

The pinhole acts as a universal correcting lens. If your vision was improved when looking through the hole, it indicates that you may need spectacles for distance vision.

When I was last at the optician's, she put drops in my eyes. Why did she do that?

These drops enlarge the pupil and make it easier for the doctor to examine the back of your eye with an ophthalmoscope. It is sometimes not possible to examine the eye properly without dilating the pupil to get a clearer view. As these drops also paralyse the lens, which allows your sight to focus properly, you should not drive immediately after leaving the clinic. The effect of the drops may last as long as 12 hours. It is worthwhile taking sunglasses with you to the clinic if they are likely to put drops in your eyes, as otherwise bright sunlight can be very uncomfortable until the drops have worn off.

Why does diabetes affect the eyes?

A simple question but difficult to answer. Current research indicates strongly that it is the excess glucose in the bloodstream that directly damages the eyes, mainly by affecting the lining of the small blood vessels that carry blood to the retina. The damage to these vessels seems to be directly proportional to how high the blood glucose is and how long it has been raised. This is the reason why we all believe that it can be avoided by bringing the blood glucose down to normal.

I have had diabetes for 20 years and seem to be quite well. When the doctor looked in my eyes at my last visit he said he could see some mild diabetic changes and referred me to a clinic called the Retinopathy Clinic. Am I about to go blind?

There is no need for alarm. It would be surprising if, after 20 years of diabetes, there were not some changes in your eyes. He probably considers it appropriate that you should be seen by an eye specialist and maybe have some special photographs taken of your eyes in order to examine them in more detail and which will be of use for future reference.

I have been diagnosed with retinopathy. Can you explain more what this is?

Retinopathy is a condition affecting the back of the eye (the retina). It may occur in people with long-standing diabetes, particularly those in whom control has not been very good. There is a gradual change in the blood vessels (arteries and veins) to the back of the eye that can lead to deterioration of vision. This may be due either to deposits in a vital area at the back of the eye or to bleeding into the eye from abnormal blood vessels.

Retinopathy is usually diagnosed by examination of the eye with an ophthalmoscope, and it can usually be picked up a long time before it leads to any disturbance in vision. Treatment at this stage with a laser usually arrests the process and slows or stops further deterioration.

On a recent TV programme it was stated that people with diabetes over 40 years of age were likely to become blind. This has horrified me because my 9-year-old son has diabetes and unfortunately some of his school friends have told him about the programme. What can I say to reassure him?

Some damage to the eyes (retinopathy) occurs quite commonly after more than 20 years of diabetes. Retinopathy is, however, usually slight and does not affect vision. Only a very small proportion of people actually go blind, probably no more than 7% of those who have had diabetes for 30 years or more. Because of the tremendous advances that have occurred in diabetes over the last 20 or 30 years, this proportion will be much less when your son has had diabetes for 30 years. The figure is likely to be smaller in people with well controlled diabetes and larger in those who are always badly controlled.

Can I wear contact lenses and if so would you recommend hard or soft ones?

The fact that you have diabetes should not interfere with your use of contact lenses or influence the sort of lens that you are given. Of greater importance in the choice of type would be local factors affecting your eyes and vision, and the correct person to advise you would be an ophthalmologist or qualified optician specializing in prescribing and fitting contact lenses. It would be sensible to let him or her know that you have diabetes and you must follow the advice given, particularly to prevent infection – but this applies to everyone, whether or not they have diabetes.

I get flashes of light and specks across my vision. Are they symptoms of serious eye trouble?

Although people with diabetes do get eye trouble, flashing lights and specks are not usually symptoms of this particular problem. You should discuss it with your own doctor who will want to examine your eyes in case there is any problem.

My father who has diabetes now has developed cataracts. Is this to with his diabetes?

Cataracts occur in people who do not have diabetes as well as in those who do, and as such are not a specific diabetic complication, although they are more common in people with diabetes. There is a very rare form of cataract that can occur in childhood with very badly controlled diabetes, known as a 'snowstorm' cataract from its characteristic appearance to the specialist. The normal common variety of cataract seen in diabetes is exactly the same as that occurring in people without diabetes, but is found at an earlier age. It is really due to the ageing process affecting the substance that makes up the lens of the eye. It develops wrinkles and becomes less transparent than normal.

Eventually it becomes so opaque that it becomes difficult to see properly through it. His doctor should arrange for your father to see an eye specialist.

The last time I was tested at the clinic, I was told that I had developed microaneurysms. What on earth are these?

Microaneurysms are little balloon-like dilatations (swellings) in the very small capillaries (blood vessels) supplying the retina at the back of the eye. They are one of the earliest signs that the high blood glucose levels seen in poorly controlled diabetes have damaged the lining to these capillaries. They do not interfere with vision as such, but give an early warning that retinopathy has begun to develop. There is some evidence to suggest that these can get better with the introduction of perfect control whereas, at later stages of diabetic retinopathy, reversal is not usually possible. Anyone who has microaneurysms must have regular eye checks, so that any serious developments are detected at an early stage. You have picked up early so now is the time to make sure that your glucose level control is impeccable!

I shall be going to have laser treatment soon on my eyes. What will this involve?

Laser treatment is a form of treatment with a narrow beam of intense light used to cause very small burns on the back of the eye (retina). It is used in the treatment of many eye conditions including diabetic retinopathy. The laser burns are made in parts of the retina not used for detailed vision, sparing the important areas required for reading, etc. This form of treatment has been shown to arrest or delay the progress of retinopathy, provided that it is given in adequate amounts at an early stage before useful vision is lost. It is sometimes necessary to give small doses of laser treatment intermittently over many years, although occasionally it can all be dealt with over a relatively short period. Your eyes will need continuous assessment thereafter, as it is possible that further treatment may be needed at any stage.

My doctor used the term 'photocoagulation' the other day. Is this the same as laser treatment? Will it damage my eyes at all?

Photocoagulation is indeed treatment of retinopathy by lasers. The strict answer as to whether it can damage your eyes is yes, but uncommonly. Occasionally the lesion produced by photocoagulation can spread and involve vital parts of the retina so that vision is affected. Normally treatment is confined to the parts of the retina that have no noticeable effect on vision other than perhaps to narrow the field of view slightly. Photocoagulation can also occasionally result in rupture of a blood vessel and haemorrhage. After a great deal of photocoagulation there is a slight risk of damage to the lens causing a type of cataract.

I have glaucoma. Is this related to diabetes?

Yes. Although glaucoma can occur quite commonly in people who do not have diabetes, there is a slightly increased risk in those who do. This is usually confined to those who have advanced diabetic eye problems (proliferative retinopathy).

Occasionally the eye drops that are put in your eyes to dilate the pupil to allow a proper view of the retina can precipitate an attack of glaucoma (increased pressure inside the eye). The signs of this would be pain in the affected eye together with blurring of vision coming on some hours after the drops have been put in. Should this occur you must seek urgent medical advice either from your own doctor or from the accident and emergency department of your local hospital. It is reversible with rapid treatment but can cause serious damage if ignored.

Every time I receive my copy of *Balance*, Diabetes UK's magazine, I have the impression that the print gets smaller. Is this true or is there something wrong with my eyes?

Eyesight tends to deteriorate with age, whether or not someone has diabetes. First you should visit your optician and get your eyesight checked to see whether it can be improved with glasses, as this may be all that is required. You should mention the fact that you have diabetes to your optician.

For people with severe retinopathy to the degree that reading becomes impossible, there are ways of helping. *Balance*, for example, is available to members of Diabetes UK as a cassette recording and this service is free of charge although, to satisfy Post Office regulations, you have to have a certificate of blindness before the cassette can be sent to you.

Public libraries can also help – most carry a wide selection of books in large type and most also lend books on cassette. Some larger libraries now have Kurtzweil machines, which can translate printed material into speech. So, in effect, they can read to you, although the 'voice' sounds a little mechanical. This can be useful for any material that you feel is confidential, such as letters, where you might not want another person to read them to you. Libraries usually have these machines in rooms of their own so, once you have been shown how to use them, you can be quite private.

The Royal National Institute for the Blind also has an excellent talking book service. *Diabetes – the 'at your fingertips' guide* is available as a talking book from the RNIB.

Feet, chiropody and footwear

I have just developed diabetes and have been warned that I am much more likely to get into trouble with my feet and need to take great care of them – what does this mean?

If you keep your diabetes well controlled, have no loss of sensation and good circulation to your feet, then you are no more at risk than a person without diabetes. In the long term people with diabetes are more likely to develop foot trouble and it pays to get into good habits – inspecting your feet daily, keeping your toenails properly trimmed and avoiding badly fitting shoes from the outset. When you have diabetes you should have access to the local NHS chiropodist (nowadays called a podiatrist), who will check your feet and advise you, free of charge, on any questions that you may have.

I have had diabetes for 10 years and as far as I can see it is quite under control and I am told that I am free from complications, but I cannot help worrying about the possibility of developing gangrene in the feet – can you tell me what it is and what causes it?

Gangrene is the death of tissues in any part of the body. It most commonly occurs in the toes and fingers. Gangrene also occurs in people without diabetes, and people with diabetes develop it only if they have a serious lack of blood supply to their feet or reduced sensation. It can also be caused by smoking, which is the main cause of clogged-up blood vessels. Generally it occurs only in older people and is related to the progressive hardening of the arteries that is part of the ageing process.

The other form of gangrene occurring in people with diabetes is caused by the presence of infection. This usually affects the feet of people who have reduced sensation because of diabetic neuropathy (see the introduction to this chapter). This can occur even in the presence of a good blood supply. Any infected break in the skin of your feet must be treated promptly and seriously. If you are worried about anything to do with your feet, then you should consult your doctor or chiropodist/podiatrist immediately.

As someone with diabetes, do I have to take any special precautions when cutting my toenails?

It is important for everyone to cut their toenails to follow the shape of the end of the toe, and not cut deep into the corners. Your toenails should not be cut too short, and you should not use any sharp instrument to clean down the sides of the nails. All this is to avoid the possibility of ingrowing toenails. If you have problems cutting your toenails consult your NHS chiropodist (podiatrist).

I have a thick callus on the top of one of my toes – can I use a corn plaster on this?

No. Do not use any corn remedies on your feet. They often contain an acid which softens the skin and increases the risk of an infection. Consult a State Registered Chiropodist to have it treated – as you have diabetes you should have access to an NHS chiropodist (podiatrist) who will treat you free of charge.

My son has picked up athlete's foot. He has diabetes treated with insulin – do I have to take any special precautions about using the powder and cream given to me by my doctor?

No. Athlete's foot is very common and is due to a fungal infection, which should respond quickly to the treatment with the appropriate antifungal preparation; this can be bought without prescription. Do not forget the usual precautions of making sure he keeps his feet clean, dries them carefully and changes his socks daily.

Will I get bunions because I have diabetes?

No. Bunions are no more common in people who have diabetes than in those who do not.

I have had diabetes for 25 years and I have been warned that the sensation in my feet is not normal. I am troubled with an ingrowing toenail on my big toe, which often gets red but does not hurt – what shall I do about it?

You should seek help and advice urgently in case it is infected. If so, you are at risk of the infection spreading without you being aware of it, because it would hurt less than in someone with normal sensation. This is potentially a serious situation, so see your doctor straight away.

I am 67 and have had diabetes for 15 years. As far as I can tell my feet are quite healthy but, as my vision is not very good, I find it difficult to inspect my feet properly – what can I do about it?

Do you have a friend or relative who could look at your feet regularly and trim your nails? If this is not possible, then the sensible thing to do would be to attend a State Registered chiropodist regularly. Ask your GP or diabetes clinic about local arrangements for seeing an NHS chiropodist (podiatrist).

Do I have to pay for chiropody?

Most hospital diabetes departments provide a chiropody (podiatry) service free of charge. Outside the hospital service, chiropody under the NHS is limited to pensioners, pregnant women and school children. Although local rules do vary, most districts consider people with diabetes as a priority group and do offer free chiropody. You should check locally before obtaining treatment. If you are seeing a chiropodist or podiatrist privately, make sure that he or she is State Registered (they will have the letters SRCh after their name).

What are the signs that diabetes may be affecting my feet?

There are two major dangers from diabetes that may affect the feet. The first is due to reduced blood supply from arterial thickening. This leads to poor circulation with cold feet, even in warm weather, and cramps in the calf when you are walking (*intermittent claudication*). This is not a specific complication of diabetes and often occurs in people who do not have diabetes. The major problem here is arterial sclerosis (hardening of the arteries), and smoking is a more important cause of this than diabetes. In severe cases this can progress to gangrene.

The second way that diabetes can affect the feet is through damage to the nerves (neuropathy), which reduces the feeling of pain and awareness of extremes of temperature. This can be quite difficult to detect unless the feet are examined by an expert.

FOOT CARE RULES

Dos

- **Do** wash your feet daily with soap and warm water. Do not use hot water – check the temperature of the water with your elbow.
- **Do** dry your feet well with a soft towel, especially between your toes.
- **Do** apply a gentle skin cream, such as E45, if your skin is rough and dry.
- **Do** change your socks or stockings daily.
- **Do** wear well-fitting shoes. Make sure they are wider, deeper and longer than your foot with a good firm fastening that you have to undo to get your foot in and out. This will prevent your foot from moving inside the shoe.
- **Do** run your hand around the inside of your shoes each day before putting them on to check that there is nothing that will rub your feet.
- **Do** wear new shoes for short periods of time and check your feet afterwards.
- **Do** cut your toenails to follow the shape of the end of your toes, not deep into the corners. This is easier after a bath as your toenails will soften in the warm water.
- **Do** check your feet daily and see your chiropodist/podiatrist or doctor about any problems.
- **Do** see a State Registered chiropodist or podiatrist if in any doubt about foot care.

Don'ts

- **Do not** put your feet on hot-water bottles or sit too close to a fire or radiator, and avoid extremes of cold and heat.
- **Do not** use corn paints or plasters or attempt to cut your own corns with knives or razors under any circumstances.
- **Do not** wear tight garters. Wear a suspender belt or tights instead.
- **Do not** neglect even slight injuries to your feet.
- **Do not** walk barefoot.
- **Do not** let your feet get dry and cracked. Use E45 or hand lotion to keep the skin soft.
- **Do not** cut your toenails too short or dig down the sides of your nails.
- **Do not** wear socks with holes in them.
- **Do not** sit with your legs crossed.
- **Do not** smoke.

FOOT CARE RULES (cont'd)

Seek advice immediately if you notice any of the following:

- Any colour change in your legs or feet.
- Any discharge from a break or crack in the skin, or from a corn or from beneath a toenail.
- Any swelling, throbbing or signs of inflammation in any part of your foot.

First aid measures

- Minor injuries can be treated at home provided that professional help is sought if the injury does not improve quickly.
- Minor cuts and abrasions should be cleaned gently with cotton wool or gauze and warm salt water. A clean dressing should be lightly bandaged in place.
- If blisters occur, do not prick them. If they burst, dress as for minor cuts.
- Never use strong medicaments such as iodine.
- Never place adhesive strapping directly over a wound: always apply a dressing first.

The danger is that any minor damage to the foot, be it from a cut or abrasion or badly fitting shoe, will not cause the usual painful reaction, so that damage can result from continued injury or infection spreading. It is important that you should know whether the sensation in your feet is normal or reduced. Make sure that you ask your doctor this at your next clinic review.

My daughter has diabetes and often walks barefoot around the house. Should I discourage her from doing this?

It is well known that people with diabetes are prone to problems with their feet which are, for the most part, due to carelessness and can be avoided. The usual reason these problems occur is that, with increasing duration of diabetes, sensation in the feet tends to be reduced. Most people are unaware of this, and so the danger is that damage to the feet may be the first indication of the problem. By then it could be too late!

The dangers to the feet of children with diabetes, however, are really very slight and there is no reason to discourage your daughter from walking about barefoot at an early age.

What special care should I take of my feet during the winter?

In older people with diabetes, the blood supply to the feet may not be as good as in those who do not have diabetes and this will make their feet more vulnerable to damage by severe cold. As winter is cold and wet, we tend to wear warmer thick clothing, and shoes, which are comfortable in the summer, may be unpleasantly tight when worn with thick woolly socks or stockings. This may damage the feet and also make them more sensitive to the cold. It could numb the sensation completely. All these effects will be made worse if your feet become wet.

Make sure your shoes are comfortable, fit well, and allow room for you to wear an adequately thick pair of socks, preferably made of wool or other absorbent material. Use weather-proof shoes, overshoes or boots if you are going to be out for any length of time in the rain or snow, and dry your feet carefully if they get wet. Do not put your cold – and slightly numb – feet straight onto a hot water bottle or near a hot fire because you may find that, when the feeling comes back, the heat is excessive and chilblains may occur. Feet also need protection during the summer as wearing open sandals can cause problems from possible damage by sharp stones, etc.

How can I give continual protection to my feet?

It is extremely difficult. If the sensation in your feet is normal, then generally you have very little need to worry but, if there is even slight numbness of your feet, you should check them daily and seek the advice of someone else to look at the areas that you have difficulty in seeing. If your circulation is poor, try hard to keep your feet warm and well protected.

FEET FACTS

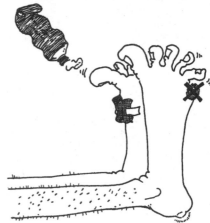

* Minor cuts or abrasions can be covered with sterile gauze after use of a mild antiseptic cream.

* Avoid using corn plasters – they contain acids which can cause problems.

* Don't prick blisters, instead treat as for a minor abrasion.

* Corns, callouses or ingrowing toenails must always be treated by your chiropodist.

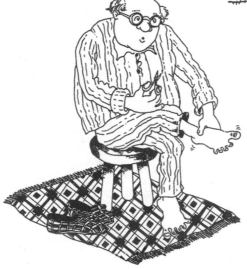

* When your toenails need cutting, always do this after bathing.

* Cut the nail edge following the shape of the end of the toe.

* Don't cut the corners of your toenails back into the nail grooves.

* Avoid using a sharp instrument to clean the free nail edge or the nail grooves.

Figure 9.1 Foot care information.

* If your skin is too dry, apply a small amount of emollient cream (e.g. E45).

* Check and bathe your feet every day, then pat dry gently, particularly between the toes.

* If your skin is moist, dab gently with surgical spirit and then dust lightly with talcum powder.

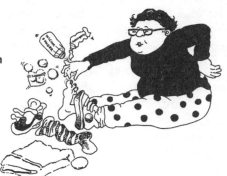

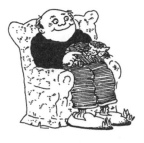

* Remove hot water bottles before getting into bed, and switch off your electric blanket.

* If thick woollen bed-socks are worn, they must be loose fitting.

* Be careful not to sit too close to radiators or fires.

* Choose shoes which provide good support. They must be broad, long and deep enough. Check that you can wriggle all your toes.

* Shoes should have a fastening.

* Check shoes daily for any small objects, such as hairpins, stones or buttons.

* If socks have ridges or seams, wear them inside out. Loose fitting ones are best.

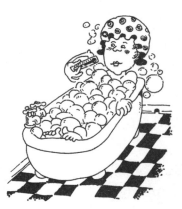

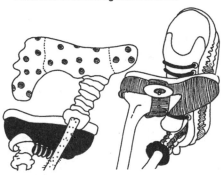

* Avoid very hot baths.

* Always dry your feet carefully after bathing.

I have suffered from foot ulcers for many years and would be grateful if you could suggest something to help my problem.

You should not attempt treatment of these yourself but you should seek medical advice and expert chiropody. Foot ulcers in people with diabetes are usually caused by reduced sensation in the feet (neuropathy) and you should have your feet examined by your specialist to find out whether this is the case. If so, you need to attend for regular chiropody and to learn all the ways of avoiding trouble once sensation is reduced. You may need special shoes made by a shoe fitter (an orthotist), which your consultant or podiatrist can arrange.

I have so many other things to remember – can you give me a simple list of rules for foot care?

The list of foot rules that we have given is aimed specifically for those who have abnormalities of either blood supply (ischaemia) or nerve damage (neuropathy). If you have poor sight then you should get somebody else with good eyesight to help you inspect and care for your feet. These 'Feet Facts' are shown in a more entertaining form in Figure 9.1!

Kidney damage

It's bad enough having diabetes. If I'm at risk also of kidney damage, what should I look for?

There are several ways in which diabetes may affect the kidneys, and they will show up in the routine urine and blood tests that you have at your diabetes clinic.

A lot of glucose in the urine puts you at risk of infection that can spread from the bladder up to the kidneys ('cystitis' and 'pyelonephritis'). Occasionally long-standing kidney infections may cause very few symptoms and are only revealed by routine tests.

People with long-standing and poorly controlled diabetes are at risk of damage to the small blood vessels supplying the kidney just as the retina of the eye may be affected. This does not produce any symptoms but will be picked up on a routine urine test carried out at the diabetes clinic. Most clinics now use a special test for detecting 'microalbuminuria', which as the name implies is a microscopic amount of albumin (protein) in the urine. This is a useful test as it can pick up the earliest signs of kidney damage.

With more severe kidney disease, large amounts of albumin may be lost in the urine. This may make the urine froth and lead to a build up of fluid in the body, which in turn leads to swelling around the ankles (oedema). Kidney failure may eventually develop in people who have had long-standing kidney problems. This is usually picked up by blood tests and urine tests years before the symptoms develop.

I have developed kidney failure. Will be possible to have dialysis or even a transplant although I have diabetes?

Yes. The majority of people who are unfortunate enough to end up with kidney failure are suitable for both forms of treatment.

Dialysis (or chronic renal replacement therapy) is of two major types. The older type is haemodialysis where the blood is washed in a special machine twice a week; the more recent is a type of dialysis known as CAPD (chronic ambulatory peritoneal dialysis) where fluid is washed in and out of the abdomen on a daily basis. People with diabetes seem to be very good at learning this method, which in some ways is simpler and cheaper than haemodialysis.

Transplantation is the aim of most dialysis programmes, but the supply of suitable kidneys is a limiting factor. The source of kidneys is from either people dying accidentally or live related donors who have agreed to give one of their two normal kidneys to a relative with kidney failure. A normal person can manage perfectly well with one kidney without any shortening of life provided that the kidney does not get damaged. The donor will, of course, have to have an operation and will be slightly more vulnerable as a result because they will have only one kidney to rely on instead of two.

I was found to have protein (albumin) in my urine when I last attended the diabetes clinic – what does this mean?

If it was only a trace of protein, it may mean nothing, but you should get your urine checked again to make sure it remains clear. If it is a consistent finding, it suggests either that you could have an infection in the bladder or kidney (cystitis or pyelonephritis) or that you have developed a degree of diabetic kidney damage (nephropathy). There are many other causes of protein (albumin) in the urine and it may not be related to your diabetes. If the protein in your urine is a consistent finding, it will need to be investigated, and you should ask to be kept informed of the results of the tests.

At my last clinic visit I was told that I had microalbumin-uria. What is this?

The very earliest stage of diabetic kidney disease leads to a leak of very small amounts of protein (albumin) into the urine. If it is a consistent finding, it suggests that your kidneys have been damaged by diabetes. If this is the case, then attention to control of your blood glucose and treatment of any tendency towards raised blood pressure is of great importance, as this can stabilize or even reverse the condition.

Nerve damage

There are various conditions that can affect the nervous system of someone with diabetes: diabetic neuritis, diabetic neuropathy, autoimmune neuropathy and diabetic amyotrophy. We discuss these below.

I have been on insulin for 3 years. Eighteen months ago I started to get pains in both legs and could barely walk. Despite treatment I am still suffering. Can you tell me what can be done to ease this pain?

There are many causes of leg pains, and only one is due specifically to diabetes. This is a particularly vicious form of *neuritis* – in other words, a form of nerve damage, which causes singularly unpleasant pain, chiefly in the feet or thighs, or sometimes both. The pain sensation is either one of pins and needles, or of constant burning, and is often worse at night causing lack of sleep. Contact from clothes or bedclothes is often acutely uncomfortable.

Fortunately this form of neuritis is rather uncommon and always disappears, although it may take many months before doing so. Very good control of your diabetes is important as it will help to alleviate the symptoms and speed their recovery. Relief is otherwise obtained by good painkillers, as recommended by your doctor, and sometimes assisted by sleeping tablets. Always remember that eventually recovery occurs, as otherwise you will find that it is easy to get despondent. Also remember that the diagnosis must be made by a doctor who will consider all the various causes of leg pains before coming to a diagnosis of diabetic neuritis.

I have had diabetes for many years but my general health is good and I am very stable. During the last year, however, I have developed an extreme soreness on the soles of my feet whenever pressure has been applied, e.g. when digging with a spade, standing on ladders, walking on hard ground or stones, even when applying the accelerator in the car. If I thump an object with the palm of my hand, I suffer the same soreness. The pain is extreme and sometimes lasts for a day or so. Could you tell me if you have heard of this condition in other people and what is the reason for it?

These symptoms may be due to diabetic neuropathy, a condition of damage to the nerves, which occasionally occurs in long-standing diabetes. It affects the feet more often than other parts of the body and often produces painful tingling or burning sensations in the feet, although numbness is perhaps more common. Strict control of your diabetes is important for the prevention and treatment of this complication – it can be made worse by moderate or high alcohol consumption.

I have diabetes controlled on diet alone. I suffer from neuritis in my face. My GP says there is no apparent reason for this but I wondered if it had anything to do with my diabetes.

Not necessarily, as there are a number of types of neuritis that can affect the face, which have absolutely nothing to do with diabetes. Examples include both shingles (herpes zoster) and Bell's palsy, although, of course, both these conditions can affect people with diabetes.

There are forms of diabetic neuritis that do affect the face: one form occasionally affects the muscles of the eye leading to double vision, while another form can cause numbness and tingling. There is also a very rare complication known as 'gustatory sweating' where sweating breaks out across the head and scalp at the start of a meal.

I have recently been told that the tingling sensation in my fingers is due to carpal tunnel syndrome and not neuropathy as was first thought. Can you please explain the difference?

In carpal tunnel syndrome (which commonly occurs in people who do not have diabetes), the nerves supplying the skin over the fingers, the palm of the hand and some of the muscles in the hand get compressed at the wrist. Occasionally injections of hydro-cortisone or related steroids into the wrist will relieve it, or it may require a small operation at the wrist to relieve the tension on the nerve. This usually brings about a dramatic relief of any pain associated with it and a recovery of sensation and muscle strength with time.

Diabetic neuropathy more commonly affects the feet than the hands and is usually a painless loss of sensation starting with the tips of the toes or fingers and moving up the legs or arms. It is only occasionally painful and may be difficult to treat. It is due to some form of generalized damage to the nerves, not to compression of any one nerve.

I have had diabetes for 27 years and have developed a complaint called bowel neuropathy. Please can you explain what this is and what the treatment is?

Bowel neuropathy is one of the features of 'autonomic neuropathy', which may occur in some people with long-standing diabetes where there is loss of function of the nerves supplying various organs in the body. In your case, the nerves that regulate the activity of your bowels have been affected. The symptoms include indigestion, occasionally vomiting, and episodes of alternating constipation and diarrhoea. Occasionally the episodes of diarrhoea are preceded by rumblings and gurglings in the stomach and sometimes this responds to a short course of antibiotics. Otherwise eating a high-fibre diet is encouraged to prevent constipation. Irritable bowel syndrome can cause symptoms not unlike this – it has nothing to do with diabetes, although it may occur in people with diabetes. If there is ever passage of blood or mucus within your stools, you should seek medical advice without delay.

The calf muscle in one leg seems to be shrinking. There is no ache and no pain. Is this anything to do with diabetes? I have been taking insulin for 30 years.

You do not mention whether you have noticed any weakness in this leg. Occasionally diabetic neuropathy can affect the nerves, which supply the muscles, in such a way that the muscle becomes weak and shrinks in size without any accompanying pain or discomfort. It sounds as if this may be your problem.

I have had diabetes for many years and have developed pain in my legs. My thighs in particular are very weak and wasted. I have been told that I have 'diabetic amyotrophy' Will it get better?

Diabetic amyotrophy is a rare condition causing pain and weakness of the legs and is due to damage to certain nerves. It usually occurs when diabetes control is very poor, but occasionally affects people with only slight elevation of the blood glucose. Strict control of diabetes leads to its improvement but it may take up to 2 years or so for it to settle. The nerves affected are those usually supplying the thigh muscles as in your case, which become wasted and get weaker.

Heart and blood vessel disease

I have read that poor circulation in the feet is a problem for people with diabetes. Is there any way I can improve my circulation to avoid developing this?

Narrowing ('hardening') of the arteries is a normal part of growing older – and the arteries to the feet can be affected by this process, leading to poor circulation in the feet and legs. This occurs in people with diabetes as well as those without, but it is more common in those who have. The causes of arterial disease are not very well understood, but we know that smoking and poor diabetes control makes it worse. So if you have diabetes and smoke cigarettes, the risk of bad circulation increases greatly. Stop smoking, control your blood glucose, and keep active – these are the only known recipes for helping the circulation.

I am in my seventies and am worried that I might develop heart problems. I am already being treated for high blood pressure. Is heart disease likely?

Heart disease is two to five times more common in people with diabetes and it goes hand in hand with high blood pressure, excess body weight and raised cholesterol. There is increasing realization that this grouping of risk factors is an important cause of premature death in diabetes. Knowing this, it is important that your blood pressure and cholesterol levels are controlled well.

My husband died recently from a heart attack. He had had diabetes for 12 years and was controlled on tablets, and at about the same time that he developed diabetes he started having angina attacks. I wondered whether these were related and whether poor control had anything to do with his fatal heart attack?

There is certainly a connection between heart disease and diabetes. It has been shown that control of high blood pressure, cholesterol, and blood glucose are effective in preventing heart disease.

I am in my early twenties, but haven't had good diabetes control for a couple of years. Will this affect my arteries in later life?

It is unlikely to have much effect but any period of poor control is not going to do any good either. Our arteries get more rigid and more clogged up as we get older and this process can be aggravated by periods of poor diabetes control and smoking.

My left leg has been amputated because I developed diabetic gangrene. I now get a lot of pain in my right foot and calf. Could too much insulin be the cause of this pain?

No. It sounds very much as if the blood supply to your leg is insufficient and that the pain in your right foot and calf is a reflection of this poor blood supply, which was the reason why you developed gangrene in your left leg. You must be very worried, particularly about the survival of your right leg. There are a number of different ways of protecting your remaining leg and these include:

- stopping smoking (if you smoke)
- keeping diabetes, blood pressure and cholesterol under very good control, and
- maintaining close contact with a podiatrist who has a special interest in diabetes.

If you do notice any sign of increased pain or change in colour, you should seek medical advice immediately.

My husband had a heart attack last year. Nine months later he had part of his leg amputated. We have been told that he could have further problems but have been given no advice. Please give us some information on what we should do to try and avoid this.

It sounds as though your husband has generalized arterial disease (arteriosclerosis) affecting his blood vessels to the heart and to the leg. There are a number of things which you and he can do that may be of help in preventing further trouble. Firstly, if he smokes, he should stop straight away; secondly, he should keep his diabetes and blood pressure as well controlled as possible; thirdly, he should keep his remaining foot and leg warm and make sure that he has expert foot care, either by a chiropodist or by you, under the supervision of a chiropodist or district nurse. If you see any signs of damage to his foot or any discolouration then seek medical advice immediately.

Blood pressure problems

Now I have been diagnosed with diabetes, will I be more prone to high blood pressure and strokes?

Yes, there seems to be a very strong link between Type 2 diabetes and high blood pressure. Unfortunately these both increase the risk of strokes. The good news is that strict control of both diabetes and blood pressure keeps down this risk. Since publication of the UKPDS findings, we realize that the blood pressure should be kept as low as 130 mmHg in diabetes.

I have been told that my blood pressure is raised as a result of diabetic kidney problems and, because of this, it is very important that I take tablets to lower it – why is this?

There is good evidence to show that lowering the blood pressure to normal in people such as yourself protects the kidneys from further damage and helps delay any further kidney problems. We also know that controlling blood pressure reduces the risk of heart disease and stroke. There have been some studies done in Germany and the UK showing that self-monitoring of blood pressure and the active participation of people in their own treatment can significantly reduce blood pressure. In the studies, people were provided with a blood pressure monitor, and were given information about high blood pressure, and non-drug remedies, such as reducing salt and increasing fruit and vegetable intake, and exercising, and were taught how to use an individual flow chart for medication. The British Hypertension Society (address in Appendix 3) provides advice on how to select a reliable monitor, and if you think that you may benefit from self-monitoring of blood pressure, you should discuss this with your health professional.

The mind

My 68-year-old mother has had diabetes for 44 years. In the past few years her mental state has deteriorated considerably and she is now difficult to manage. Is this common for someone who has been on insulin for so long?

Memory loss (most commonly Alzheimer's disease) is mainly a problem of the elderly. People are also more likely to develop diabetes as they get older, so it is likely that both these problems may sometimes affect the same person. There is some disturbing evidence that memory loss may be more common in old people with diabetes than those without. However, the extra risk in diabetes is only small, and we do not know the relevant importance of other factors such as smoking and high blood pressure. So it is possible, but not certain, that your mother's memory problem is related to diabetes.

I had a brain haemorrhage 18 months ago and I have had diabetes since childhood. Am I more likely to get complications from diabetes?

Brain haemorrhages and strokes are more common in people with diabetes than in those without, particularly if blood pressure levels are high. Your treatment is no different than from anyone else with your condition. Your doctor will be on the lookout for chest infections and pneumonia, particularly if you have any problems with swallowing.

I have been very depressed since my diagnosis. Are people with diabetes more prone to depression or suicide, or other psychiatric illnesses?

There is some evidence to suggest that people with diabetes are prone to depression, and the suicide rate is higher than in the general population. This is probably due to the demands of a long-term condition that has an impact on daily living rather than a result of the diabetes itself. Recent studies have found that the tendency to depression can be helped by letting people become more involved in the management of their diabetes. You have obviously taken a first step in recognizing that you have depression. Visit your doctor to discuss how you feel. There is help out there!

I have read that hypos can cause brain damage – is this true?

The strict answer is yes, but only very occasionally. Only a severe hypo causing a long period of unconsciousness can lead to brain damage and this is extremely unusual. There is no evidence to suggest that the repeated hypos, which may be common in people taking insulin, cause any permanent brain damage.

10

Research and the future

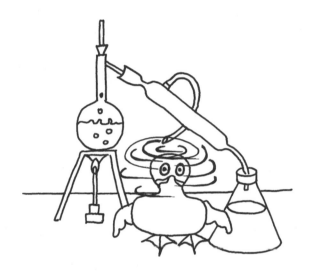

New developments and improvements in existing treatments can occur only through research; therefore research is vital to every person with diabetes. In the UK, Diabetes UK spends large sums each year (more than £4.9 million in 2000) on research into diabetes; similar large amounts of money are contributed by the Medical Research Council, the Wellcome Trust and other grant-giving bodies. The more money that is raised for research into diabetes, the greater the benefits to the population with diabetes. At the time of writing, it costs about £40,000 to support a relatively junior research worker for just 1 year. The discovery of insulin was made by a doctor and a medical student (Banting and Best) doing research together for just one summer (1921). There have been many important but less dramatic discoveries since then, each in some way contributing to our understanding of diabetes and many improving the available treatment.

Look at the Diabetes UK website for details of Diabetes UK research activities (see Appendix 3).

Searching for causes and cures

Do you think that diabetes will ever be cured?

This question cannot be answered – yet. We must always try to take an optimistic view, however, and, if diabetes cannot yet be cured, it is not for want of research. Not only does Diabetes UK have meetings to discuss research and progress, but there is also an annual European Association for the Study of Diabetes meeting and an International Diabetes Federation congress which meets every third year. In addition there are also a great many national organizations that meet regularly. More has been discovered during the last 30 years about the cause of diabetes than ever before, and during the same period there have been important advances in treatment. This is therefore a very exciting period in diabetes research and we can continue to look forward to improvements in our understanding of the disease even if, for the moment, a cure is a little too much to hope for.

I have a friend who has been treated with insulin for 12 years. He recently came off insulin altogether after having had an operation on his adrenal gland. He now tells me that his diabetes has been cured. I thought there was no cure for diabetes.

It sounds as if your friend was one of the very few people in whom the diabetes was secondary to some other condition. In his case the other condition was an adrenal tumour. When this was eventually diagnosed and appropriately treated by an operation, it resulted in a cure for his diabetes. This result has been recorded in two forms of adrenal tumour. One is called a 'phaeochromocytoma', where the tumour produces adrenaline and noradrenaline, both of which inhibit insulin secretion by the pancreas. The other adrenal tumour is one producing excess of adrenal steroids and cortisone, which again produces a form of diabetes reversible on removal of the tumour.

There are a number of other rare conditions often associated with disturbances of other hormone-producing glands in the body. In these cases cure of diabetes is possible after appropriate therapy of the hormonal disturbance. Unfortunately, less than 1% of all people with diabetes, who have such a hormonal imbalance, are suitable for surgery. Specialists are always on the lookout for these causes since the benefits from an operation are so tremendous.

Will it ever be possible to prevent diabetes with a vaccine?

There is some evidence to suggest that certain virus infections can cause diabetes but we are not clear how often this happens: it is probably very infrequently. If a virus were isolated, which was found to cause diabetes, it would then be possible to produce a vaccine that could be given to children like the polio vaccine, to prevent them from developing diabetes later in life. At present this possibility seems rather remote.

Genetics

I gather that it is possible to identify people by looking at special blood tests within a family who are at high risk of developing diabetes. This sounds like an exciting development, as presumably children who have inherited an increased risk of diabetes will be those most in need of vaccination should a vaccine become available.

Yes, you are quite right. Studies of the so-called HLA tissue antigens in families in whom there appears to be a lot of diabetes, indicate that certain patterns of inherited antigens carry with them the susceptibility to diabetes. With these tissue markers (discovered by using blood tests) it should be possible to identify the children who are likely to benefit most from a vaccine or an effective form of preventive treatment should one become available in the future. It will be in these susceptible individuals that the first clinical trials will need to be done.

Is it true that studying families who have several members with diabetes can help find a cure for the condition?

Family studies are very important for helping to understand the inheritance of diabetes. In some families there is a clear association between a certain genetic background and the development of diabetes. Some members who have not yet developed diabetes may have the 'markers' described in the answer to the previous question, indicating that they are at increased risk of developing the condition.

Is it possible to prevent diabetes in these high-risk people?

Diabetes has a genetic link and close relatives of people with the condition have an increased chance of developing it, i.e. they are 'high risk'. There is a trial taking place in the USA and Canada called the Diabetes Prevention Trial-Type 1, which is looking at people who are at high risk for Type 1 diabetes, and seeing if intervention can prevent or delay Type 1 diabetes. The participants have a test to see if their blood contains islet cell antibodies (ICA), the antibodies that destroy the insulin-producing cells, and, if they do, they are possible recruits for the trial. Over a 5-year period, these individuals either inject low doses of insulin twice a day, or take insulin orally in the form of a capsule (or are part of a control group where no insulin is given). The insulin capsules are made up of insulin crystals, which are thought to be effective against the islet cell antibodies, but are not effective for controlling the condition after onset. Animal research and studies in humans have suggested that diabetes can be delayed in those at high risk when they are given small doses of insulin. The results of the trial should be interesting.

I have heard that there is a new programme called DAFNE. What does it involve? Could I take part?

DAFNE stands for Dose Adjustment For Normal Eating. It is an educational programme, first developed in Germany, aimed at people with Type 1 diabetes, which teaches them how to adjust their insulin injections to fit their life and food patterns, rather than the other way around. The intensive course takes place over a 5-day period, and is run by specialist diabetes nurses and dietitians, and about eight people with diabetes take part. They have to take several insulin injections a day, as well as monitoring blood glucose levels at least four times a day. It teaches them how to count carbohydrate units and to adjust their insulin to their individual lifestyle, whilst keeping their blood glucose levels controlled. Results suggest that, for the right sort of person, DAFNE is a liberating experience and that the freedom to eat what you want improves the enjoyment of life. As DAFNE develops, more centres will be involved. A similar lifestyle programme for Type 2 diabetes, DESMOND, is under development. For further information speak to a member of your diabetes team, or contact the Careline (see Appendix 3).

Transplantation

I should like to volunteer to have a pancreas transplant. Is there someone I must apply to? How successful have these operations been?

Pancreatic transplantation is still in the experimental stages and it will be difficult to find anyone who will accept you as a volunteer. Technically, pancreatic transplants are even more difficult than liver, kidney or heart transplants. The pancreas is very delicate and, as the seat of many digestive juices, has a tendency to digest itself if damaged even slightly. The duct or passageway through which these juices pass is narrow, and has to be joined up to the intestines in a very intricate way so that the enzymes do not leak. Even if everything goes well technically, the body will still react against transplant so several immunosuppressant drugs have to be given. Some of these (particularly steroids), given in high doses to suppress rejection of the transplant tend to cause diabetes or make existing diabetes worse! The future looks much more promising with the transplant of the islet cells of the pancreas (see next question).

Are there any hospitals carrying out transplants of the islets of Langerhans? Would I be able to donate my cells to my insulin-treated daughter?

Yes, there are seven centres around the UK that have signed up to the Diabetes UK Islet Transplantation Consortium. This consortium is hoping to replicate and refine the technique developed by the English surgeon, James Shapiro, and his team in Edmonton, Canada. The Edmonton team took islet cells from donor pancreases and injected them into the liver of people with Type 1 diabetes. Once in the liver the cells developed a blood supply and began producing insulin. The entire transplantation process is now known as the 'Edmonton Protocol'.

However, it is not possible to take islets from living donors so you would be unable to donate your cells to your daughter. This technique is still in the experimental stage but the results look promising. In Edmonton, 13 out of 15 islet cell transplants have been 100% successful, but until the people have lived with the transplants for a number of years it is difficult to know whether this can be seen as a cure.

Transplant of the islets of Langerhans still involves the use of drugs to prevent rejection of the new cells (immunosuppressive therapy), and as result only people who have extreme problems in controlling their blood glucose levels are being considered for transplantation. People who receive islet cell transplantations spend the rest of their lives taking immunosuppressive drugs, and the long-term effects of taking these drugs are not yet known and may be damaging.

Research into 'microencapsulation' of these islets is making some progress, and may one day offer a solution that will avoid lifelong immunosuppressive therapy. By enclosing the islets in a porous membrane and transplanting them into an animal with diabetes, it is possible to show that the insulin can get out of the 'bag of islets' and normalize the blood glucose at the same time as nutrients from the bloodstream can get in to sustain the islets – while this is going on the membrane keeps at bay the cells responsible for tissue rejection. Unfortunately, after a while, the membrane tends to get clogged with scar tissue and the islet graft stops working.

A few years ago there was excitement in the media about an article in the medical journal, *The Lancet*, reporting a successful transplant of encapsulated islets. The man who received the transplant was still being treated with immunosuppressant drugs as he had received a kidney transplant as well. This result was encouraging, but much more research still has to be done before this could be considered as a form of treatment for diabetes.

Until there has been a major breakthrough in the transplantation of tissues from one individual to another, the hazards of long-term immunosuppressive therapy for someone receiving either a pancreas transplant or an islet cell transplant are greater than those of having diabetes treated with insulin. There are no tangible benefits yet for this form of therapy as a primary form of treatment for diabetes. The problems are not insuperable but much more research needs to be done before transplantation becomes a routine treatment for diabetes.

Insulin pumps and artificial pancreas

I recently read about a device called a 'glucose sensor', which can control the insulin administered to animals with diabetes. Will this ever be used on humans and if so what can we expect from it?

The research into the development of a small electronic device that could be implanted under the skin and that could continuously monitor the level of glucose in the blood has been going on in the USA, the UK and several other countries for many years. The technical problems of such a device are, however, considerable, and it seems unlikely to be of use in people with diabetes for at least some time. Not only are there technical problems in achieving an accurate reflection of blood glucose level by such a subcutaneous implanted glucose sensor, but the further problem of 'hooking it up' to a supply of insulin to be released according to the demand is formidable. Clinical trials are being carried out in the USA and France using an intravenous glucose sensor in conjunction with an implantable pump. The early results are encouraging, but it will be several years before it is widely available.

I understand that there are ways of testing blood glucose without pricking the skin. Can you tell me more about them?

There are regular reports in the press about 'non-invasive' blood glucose monitoring devices being developed. Some devices being developed are not totally non-invasive. One involves a needle being inserted under the skin for up to 3 days at a time so that blood glucose readings can be taken every few minutes. At the moment the readings given can be accessed only by a healthcare professional, but it is hoped that eventually people would be able to read these results for themselves. This method of monitoring could be useful if the device were attached to an insulin pump adjusting the amount of insulin administered in response to the blood glucose level. Although this is not yet possible, it is likely to be developed in the very near future.

The other non-invasive blood glucose monitoring device is the GlucoWatch, developed by a Californian company called Cygnus Inc. This device is worn like a wristwatch and measures blood glucose from interstitial fluid. Interstitial fluid is the fluid that fills blisters when skin is damaged, and it can be extracted from the top layers of skin without the use of a lancet. It works by a process called reverse iontophoresis. This means that a very low electric current is applied to draw interstitial fluid through the skin. The glucose in the fluid is then collected in a gel that is part of the AutoSensor, which gives a glucose measurement. The AutoSensors must be replaced every 12 hours, and the device then needs a 3-hour warm-up period. The device must be calibrated against a finger-prick blood test each time a new AutoSensor is used. The readings are taken up to three times an hour. It has a memory that can store up to 4000 results. It is recommended that people do not alter medication based on a GlucoWatch result without checking this against a finger prick test. It is now available in the UK from Cygnus (UK) Ltd, but it is expensive (contact Cygnus for information – see Appendix 3). Diabetes UK Careline can provide an information sheet on the product.

I hear that there are pumps available that can be implanted like pacemakers – is this true? What are the likely developments with insulin pumps within the next 5 years?

Yes, it is true that insulin pumps have been implanted into people as part of research studies and there has been some encouraging progress in this field. Although still experimental and with a long time to go before being a regular form of treatment, some pumps have been developed that are small enough to be implanted into the muscles forming the wall of the abdomen and have been left there for several years. The implantable pump is licensed for sale in Europe but is currently not available in the UK, and it has not been approved by the FDA in the USA. It is made by MiniMed and is very expensive. This pump does not have a sensor to detect glucose; it simply infuses insulin at a slow rate that can be regulated from the outside using a small radio transmitter. This can be used to command the pump to infuse more insulin just before a meal, or to reduce the rate of infusion if the blood glucose readings are too low. The pump has a reservoir of insulin that can be refilled with a syringe and needle, through the skin, without too much trouble, but changing the batteries requires an operation! Although it looks promising, the major disadvantages are cost and complexity. This is still very much a research procedure and cannot yet be recommended for routine treatment.

I have heard about the artificial pancreas or 'Biostator'. Apparently this machine is capable of maintaining blood glucose at normal levels, irrespective of what is eaten. Is this true? If so, why isn't it widely available?

There are several versions of what you describe, namely an artificial pancreas, which measure the glucose concentration in the bloodstream continuously and infuse insulin in sufficient quantities to keep the blood glucose normal. Unfortunately these machines are technically very complex, bulky and extremely expensive. Their major value is for research purposes since they are quite unsuitable at present as devices for long-term control.

There is a great deal of research going on in several bio-engineering groups to try and make them the same size as a cardiac pacemaker, but it is still likely to be several years before the first machines become available for research studies, and it will be a long time after that before suitably reliable machines are available for daily treatment. Even when the technical problems have been resolved and it has been miniaturized to an acceptable size for implantation, the costs are likely to be a limiting factor.

New insulin and oral insulin

What advances can we expect in the development of new insulin in the coming years?

Over the last 20 years we have gone through a stage of producing purer and purer insulins with patterns of absorption varying from the very quick-acting to the very long-acting formulations. In recent times biosynthetic human insulins have replaced the animal insulins for most people. We go into more detail about human insulins in Chapter 3, but basically they are manufactured by interfering with the genetic codes of bacteria and yeasts and inserting material that 'instructs' the organisms to produce insulin. By inserting the genetic material coding for human insulin, scientists can get the organisms to produce human insulin. They can equally well get them to make any insulin with a known structure; indeed, they can even get them to make 'new' insulins with 'invented' structures – we are now in the era of 'designer' insulins! There is virtually unlimited capability to modify the natural insulin and see if we can improve on this: by analogy to other areas, we expect to be able to develop a whole new range of insulins with new properties that should be able to make therapy better.

We are already beginning to see the benefits from this remarkable advance in scientific manufacturing. Trials have shown that one of these insulins is absorbed much more quickly than any of the existing fast-acting insulins, is very good for covering meals and can be given immediately before the meal rather that 15–30 minutes beforehand. Two such insulins have now been released for general use, Humalog from Lilly and Novorapid from NovoNordisk (see Table 3.1 in Chapter 3).

We are also looking for variations in the structure of the insulin, which will 'target' the insulin more directly to the liver, the major organ responsible for glucose production in the body. Normally insulin is produced by the pancreas and goes directly to the liver but, unfortunately, in insulin-treated people, the injected insulin reaches the liver only after it has been through all the other tissues in the body. It should be possible to modify the structure in such a way that it can be targeted at the liver and in that way, perhaps, it may turn out to be a more effective and easier way of controlling blood glucose levels.

I have heard that it is possible to get away from insulin injections either by using nasal insulin sprays or some form of insulin that is active when taken by mouth. Are these claims true and are we going to be able to get away from insulin injections in the future?

There is no doubt that a small proportion of any insulin delivered via the **nose** is absorbed through the membranes into the bloodstream and can lower the blood glucose. Unfortunately only a small percentage of that which is put into the nose is ever absorbed and it is therefore an inefficient and expensive way of administering insulin. Because the absorption is erratic, the blood glucose is not very stable. Experiments have been done with insulin suppositories showing that they too can lower the blood glucose without the need for injections but, again, the absorption is only incomplete and the response erratic.

Regarding **oral insulins**, it is possible to prevent the stomach from digesting the insulin by incorporating it into a fat (lipid) droplet (liposome), which enables it to be absorbed from the gut without being broken down by the digestive juices. Unfortunately again, the absorption is erratic, the whole lipid droplet with the insulin is absorbed, and there is no way of knowing when the insulin will be released from the droplet and become active.

Inhale Therapeutic Systems Inc. is developing an **insulin inhaler** (using compressed air), that delivers an insulin powder deep into the lungs, where it is absorbed into the bloodstream, (a pulmonary drug delivery system). These new forms of insulin are taking a long time to come onto the market and we just have to wait and see how successful they will be. NovoNordisk and Aradigm Corporation are beginning further trials of their insulin inhaler. This is an electronic inhaler that releases a blister pack of liquid insulin deep into the lungs. Generex Biotechnology Corporation is developing an oral insulin spray administered by a device that looks like a small asthma inhaler. A pressurised container holding liquid insulin administers the drug into the mouth, and this is quickly absorbed through the cheeks into the bloodstream.

Oral **insulin crystals** are being used in capsule form in the Diabetes Prevention Trial in the USA (see a previous question in this chapter), but, although they are thought to be effective against the antibodies that destroy the insulin-producing cells, they cannot control the diabetes after onset.

All these developments are exciting but there are various issues to be aware of when considering the effectiveness of inhaled and oral insulin:

- People must be confident of receiving an accurate dose of the insulin.
- Inhalers often use very large doses of insulin.
- We do not yet know the potential side effects of such large doses.
- The inhalers being developed so far do not totally eliminate the need for insulin injections.
- The devices need to be portable, compact and competitively priced.

We await the publication of the clinical trials with great interest. Diabetes UK is likely to keep people informed by articles in *Balance*, or on their website.

New technology

Will there be any benefits to people with diabetes from the computer and microelectronic revolution?

You will have already seen some of the benefits in the blood glucose monitoring devices currently available, and all the modern insulin pumps rely heavily on microchips to control the rate of infusion.

We have microcomputer programs that help store and analyse home blood glucose monitoring records. It should be possible soon to simulate the blood glucose response to different insulin injections and in this way produce means of exploring the effect of different types and doses of insulin, and simulating the body's response. We are also using computers as a way of teaching people about diabetes and its management, as well as a way of testing people about their knowledge of diabetes. There is now a multimedia interactive CD ROM containing a great deal of excellent educational material but, as it is expensive at present, it is only suitable for diabetes clinic or practice use. Microcomputers are being used to help record and analyse information from the diabetes clinic as well as to help to plan and organize monitoring of diabetes care and to write letters. It is quite likely that this will lead to an improvement in the efficiency of the organization of diabetes clinics, as it has done to the organizing, for example, of airline tickets and flights. There are early experiments going on in the use of so-called 'expert systems' to transfer the expert knowledge and reasoning of specialists to general practitioners in order to facilitate their management of people with diabetes within general practice, without the need for them to attend hospital diabetes clinics so often.

It is not unreasonable to expect that the microelectronic revolution will produce a lot of benefits over the next 10 years.

Our local diabetes unit has just run a successful Christmas Fair to raise a lot of money for a mass spectrometer. What good is this going to do for diabetes research?

A mass spectrometer is a complicated machine, which can be used to measure minute amounts of very similar substances present in the bloodstream or in other body constituents. It is often used to measure the amounts of naturally occurring stable 'isotopes', which can be administered to people with diabetes to investigate their body's metabolism in great detail. In the past this type of study could be done only by injecting radioactive isotopes, which could then be followed in the body as they were metabolized. As their name implies, radioisotopes produce radiation, which can have harmful effects on cells in the body. As we know, even the smallest amount of radiation is best avoided: mass spectrometry allows even more detailed research into metabolism than radioisotopes with none of the risk. Your local researchers are lucky to have this facility.

11
Self-help groups

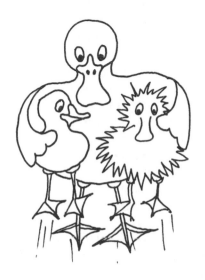

This chapter is about the various organizations that have grown up to help their members. It is a straightforward description of what is available and is not written as questions and answers.

People react in different ways to the shock of diabetes: some try to become hermits and hide, while others set out to try to solve all the problems of mankind (including diabetes) in a few weeks. Whatever your reaction, you should make contact with your local Diabetes UK group. You will come across people who are living with diabetes and who have learnt to cope with many of the daily problems. These people should provide an extra dimension to the information that you have been given by doctors, nurses, dietitians and other professionals.

Diabetes UK

This was founded in 1934, under the name of the British Diabetic Association by two people with diabetes, H. G. Wells, the author, and R. D. Lawrence, a doctor based at the diabetes clinic of King's College Hospital, London. In a letter to *The Times* dated January 1933, they announced their intention to set up an 'Association open to all diabetics, rich or poor, for mutual aid and assistance, and to promote the study, the diffusion of knowledge, and the proper treatment of diabetes in this country'. They proposed that people with diabetes, members of the general public interested in diabetes, and doctors and nurses should be persuaded to join the projected association. Nearly 70 years later Diabetes UK is a credit to its founders.

It has more than 190,000 members, and an annual budget in excess of £16 million. In many countries there are separate organizations for people with diabetes and for professionals, but Diabetes UK draws its strength from the fact that both interest groups are united in the same society. Diabetes UK is the largest organization in the UK working for people with diabetes, funding research, campaigning, and helping people live with the condition. The Careline (020 7424 1030, Monday–Friday, 9am–5pm) offers confidential support and information on all aspects of diabetes. During 2000 Careline handled in excess of 47,000 queries. In order to make Careline accessible to all, there is access to an interpreting service.

Many people with diabetes experience discrimination in terms of increased premiums, restricted terms or even can have policies refused when taking out insurance. Faced with the general lack of understanding within the insurance market, Diabetes UK has negotiated its own exclusive schemes to provide policies suited to the needs of people with diabetes and those living with them. Diabetes UK Services offers competitively priced home and motor, travel and personal finance products. For details of home, travel and motor insurance, as well as personal finance, telephone 0800 731 7431 (or e-mail *diabetes@heathlambert.com*).

Up to date information and news is published in *Balance*, a magazine that appears every other month. *Diabetes for beginners* is provided for newly diagnosed people, both Type 1 and Type 2 (insulin dependent and non-insulin dependent). Diabetes UK produces its own handbooks, leaflets and videotapes for teaching purposes, and also sells those produced by other publishers. It constantly lobbies for high standards of care for those with diabetes. Diabetes UK has an excellent website. Diabetes UK's address and website address is given in Appendix 3.

Diabetes UK organizes 'living with diabetes' days. These are one-day conferences for people with diabetes, their carers, families and friends, giving an opportunity to talk to healthcare professionals and people living with diabetes, and to discover more about Diabetes UK. For more information contact the conference team at Diabetes UK, telephone 020 7424 1000.

Diabetes UK holidays

The first diabetes holidays for children in the UK took place in 1935 and these have grown into a large enterprise. During the summer of 2000, at 12 different sites throughout the UK, 500 children, aged between 7–18 years, enjoyed a week away with Diabetes UK. These educational holidays are organized by the care interventions team, and they give the opportunity for children to meet others with diabetes and to become more independent of their parents. They aim to give the children a good time, and encourage them to try new activities, whilst teaching them more about their diabetes and to provide a well-earned break for their parents.

Diabetes UK family weekends

The care intervention team also organizes family weekends for parents of children with diabetes. These cater for about 200 families each year. While parents have talks and discussions from specialist doctors, nurses and dietitians, there are activities for children throughout the weekend supervised by skilled and experienced helpers.

Youth Education Project

This project encourages locally organized educational events. In 2000 about 700 children took part in one of 28 events. Each event received a grant from Diabetes UK, and additional support in the form of guidelines and advice.

Local Diabetes UK branches

There are over 430 branches and parents' groups throughout the country. These are run entirely by volunteers and, because of their commitment, large sums of money are raised for research into diabetes. Diabetes UK branches also aim to increase public awareness of diabetes, and arrange meetings for local people with diabetes and their families for support and information.

Parent support groups

Parents of young children with diabetes often feel they have special needs – and that they can offer particular help to other parents in the same boat. Over 80 parent support groups exist throughout the UK and they have added a sense of urgency to the main aim of Diabetes UK: to improve the lives of people with diabetes and to work towards a future without diabetes. In addition to self-help, the parents' groups also raise money for research.

The care intervention team now runs a 'Parent-link', which is a network support system for parents of children with diabetes that aims to put parents in touch from a gradually expanding database. Parent-link sends out a newsletter called *Link-Up* four times a year.

Joining Diabetes UK

Diabetes UK works to influence the decisions made about living with diabetes, and the more members it has, the greater its influence. Diabetes UK cannot continue to provide its services and activities to all people with diabetes without your support. If you would like more information about joining Diabetes UK, contact the Supporter Development department on 0207 323 1531 or write to Diabetes UK at the address shown in Appendix 3.

Diabetes UK's Necrobiosis Support Network

This enables people with necrobiosis to get in touch with others with the condition. Contact the Careline (see Appendix 3).

Tadpole Club

This is a club for younger children with diabetes, their families and friends, which sends out a regular fun newsletter called the *Tadpole Times*. More information (including current membership fee) can be obtained from Diabetes UK (address in Appendix 3).

Juvenile Diabetes Research Foundation (JDRF)

This organization was founded in 1970 by a small group of parents of children with diabetes. The Juvenile Diabetes Research Foundation exists to find a cure for diabetes and its complications. They support diabetes worldwide and provide research funds at a comparable level to Diabetes UK. The address and website can be found in Appendix 3.

Insulin Pump Therapy Group

This group was formed to raise funds and provide information on insulin pumps. The address and website can be found in Appendix 3.

Insulin Dependent Diabetes Trust (IDDT)

This is a registered charity formed in 1994, which is concerned with listening to the needs of people who live with diabetes. The aims of the Trust are:

- to offer care and support to people with diabetes and their carers, especially those experiencing difficulties with genetically engineered 'human' insulin;
- to influence appropriate bodies to ensure that a wide range of insulins remains available, to ensure that all insulin users have a continued supply of their chosen insulin;
- to ensure that all people with diabetes and carers are properly informed of the various treatments available to them, as is their right under *The Patients' Charter*;
- to collect information and experiences from people with diabetes and their carers to help others in the same situation and to pass it to healthcare professionals to create a better understanding of 'life with diabetes';
- where possible, to represent the direct voice of the person with diabetes, as the consumer, in relation to health care and research.

The Trust is run entirely by voluntary donations and does not accept funding from the pharmaceutical industry, in order to remain uninfluenced and independent. The address and website can be found in Appendix 3.

12
Emergencies

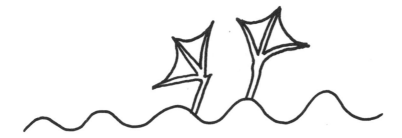

This chapter is for quick reference if things are going badly wrong. It includes vital information for people with diabetes themselves, as well as some simple rules for relatives and friends. They are designed to be consulted in an emergency, although it would be well worth your checking through them before you reach crisis point. It seems a pity to end this book in such a negative way by telling you what to do in a crisis. We hope that by keeping your diabetes well controlled you will avoid these serious situations.

What every person on insulin must know

- NEVER stop insulin if you feel ill or sick. Check your blood sugar – you may need extra insulin even if you are not eating very much.

- If you are being sick, try to keep up a good fluid intake – at least 2½ litres (4 pints) a day. If you are vomiting and unable to keep down fluids, you probably need to go to hospital for an intravenous drip.

- ALWAYS CARRY SUGAR or some similar quick-acting carbohydrate on your person.

- NEVER risk driving if your blood sugar could be low. People with diabetes DO lose their driving licences if found at the wheel when hypo.

- REMEMBER physical exercise and alcohol are both likely to bring on a hypo.

What other people must know about diabetes

- NEVER stop insulin in case of sickness (no apologies for repeating this).

- Repeated vomiting, drowsiness and laboured breathing are bad signs in someone with diabetes. They suggest impending coma and can be treated ONLY in hospital.

- A person who is hypo may not be in full command of his or her senses and may take a lot of persuasion to have some sugar. Jam or a sugary drink (e.g. Lucozade) may be easier to get down than Dextro-energy tablets. Hypostop, a glucose gel, may be useful.

- NEVER let someone drive if you suspect they are hypo. It could be fatal.

Foods to eat in an emergency or when feeling unwell

Each of the following contains 10 g carbohydrate:

- 100 ml pure fruit juice
- 100 ml Coca-Cola (*not* Diet Coke)
- 60 ml Lucozade
- Small scoop ice-cream
- 2 sugar cubes or 2 teaspoons of sugar
- 1 ordinary jelly cube or 2 heaped tablespoons of made-up jelly
- ⅓ pint (approx. 200 ml) of milk
- Small bowl of thickened soup
- 2 cream crackers
- 1 natural yogurt
- 1 diet fruit yogurt
- 1 apple or pear or orange
- 1 small banana
- 3 Dextro-energy tablets

If you are feeling unwell, eating solid foods may not be possible and you may need to rely on sweet fluids to provide the necessary carbohydrate. Liquids such as cold, defizzed (i.e. allowed to stand and go flat) Coca-Cola or Lucozade are useful if you feel sick. Do not worry about eating the exact amount of carbohydrate at the correct time but take small amounts often.

If you continue to vomit, SEEK MEDICAL ADVICE.

Signs and symptoms of hypoglycaemia and hyperglycaemia

Hypoglycaemia

This is LOW blood sugar. Also called a hypo, a reaction or an insulin reaction. Signs and symptoms include:

- FAST onset

- Tingling of the lips and tongue
- Weakness
- Tiredness
- Sleepiness
- Trembling
- Hunger
- Blurred vision
- Palpitation
- Nausea
- Headache
- Sweating
- Mental confusion
- Stumbling
- Pallor
- Slurred speech
- Bad temper
- Change in behaviour
- Lack of concentration
- Unconsciousness (hypoglycaemic or insulin coma).

Hyperglycaemia

This is HIGH blood sugar. Signs and symptoms include:

- SLOW onset (usually more than 24 hours)
- Thirst
- Excess urine
- Nausea
- Abdominal pain
- Vomiting
- Drowsiness
- Rapid breathing
- Flushed, dry skin
- Unconsciousness (hyperglycaemic or diabetic coma).

Glossary

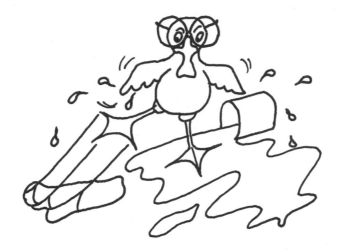

Terms in *italics* in these definitions refer to other terms in the glossary.

acarbose A drug that slows the digestion and absorption of complex carbohydrates.

Acesulfane-K A low-calorie intense sweetener.

acetone One of the chemicals called *ketones* formed when the body uses up fat for energy. The presence of acetone in the urine usually means that more insulin is needed.

adrenaline A hormone produced by the adrenal glands, which prepares the body for action (the 'flight or fight' reaction) and also causes an increase in blood glucose levels. Produced by the body as a result of many stimuli including when the blood glucose falls too low.

albumin A protein present in most animal tissues. The presence of albumin in the urine may denote kidney damage or just simply a urinary infection.

alpha cell The cell that produces *glucagon* – found in the *islets of Langerhans* in the *pancreas.*

alpha glucosidase inhibitor A tablet that slows the digestion of carbohydrates in the intestine (acarbose).

analogue insulin Insulin that has the molecular structure changed to alter the action of the insulin.

antigens Protein substances, which the body recognizes as 'foreign' and which trigger an immune response.

arteriosclerosis or **arterial sclerosis** or **arterial disease** Hardening of the arteries. Loss of elasticity in the walls of the arteries from thickening and calcification. Occurs with advancing years in those with or without diabetes. May affect the heart, causing thrombosis, or affect the circulation, particularly in the legs and feet.

aspartame A low-calorie intense sweetener. Brand name NutraSweet.

autonomic neuropathy Damage to the system of nerves that regulate many autonomic functions of the body such as stomach emptying, sexual function (potency) and blood pressure control.

bacteria A type of germ.

balanitis Inflammation of the end of the penis, usually caused by yeast infections resulting from the presence of sugar in the urine.

beef insulin Insulin extracted from the *pancreas* of cattle.

beta-blockers Drugs that block the effect of stress hormones on the cardiovascular system. Often used to treat angina and to lower blood pressure. May change the warning signs of *hypoglycaemia.*

beta cell The cell that produces insulin – found in the *islets of Langerhans* in the *pancreas.*

biguanides A group of antidiabetes tablets that lower blood glucose levels. They work by increasing the uptake of glucose by muscle, by reducing the absorption of glucose by the intestine and by reducing the amount of glucose produced by the liver. The only preparation in this group is metformin.

blood glucose monitoring System of measuring blood glucose levels at home using special reagent sticks and a special meter.

bran Indigestible husk of the wheat grain. A type of *dietary fibre*.

brittle diabetes Term used to refer to diabetes that is very unstable with swings from very low to very high blood glucose levels.

calories Units in which energy or heat are measured. The energy value of food is measured in calories.

carbohydrates A class of food that comprises starches and sugars and is most readily available by the body for energy. Found mainly in plant foods. Examples are rice, bread, potatoes, pasta, beans.

cataract Opacity of the lens of the eye, which obscures vision. It may be removed surgically.

clear insulin Soluble or regular insulin.

cloudy insulin Longer-acting insulin with fine particles of insulin bound to protamine or zinc.

coma A form of unconsciousness from which people can only be roused with difficulty. If caused by diabetes, may be a *diabetic coma* or an *insulin coma*.

complications Long-term consequences of imperfectly controlled diabetes. For details see Chapter 9.

control Usually refers to blood glucose control. The aim of good control is to achieve normal blood glucose levels (4–10 mmol/l).

coronary heart disease Disease of the blood vessels supplying the heart.

cystitis Inflammation of the bladder causing frequency of passing urine and a burning sensation when passing urine.

DAFNE Stands for Dose Adjustment For Normal Eating. An intensive education programme for learning how to match the dose of insulin to food intake and exercise.

detemir A new insulin analogue designed to last for 24 hours and act as basal insulin. Also called Levemir.

Dextro-Energy Glucose tablets.

diabetes insipidus A disorder of the pituitary gland accompanied by excessive urination and thirst. Nothing to do with *diabetes mellitus*.

diabetes mellitus A disorder of the *pancreas* characterized by a high blood glucose level. This book is about diabetes mellitus.

diabetic amyotrophy Rare condition causing pain and/or weakness of the legs from the damage to certain nerves.

diabetic coma Extreme form of *hyperglycaemia*, usually with *ketoacidosis*, causing unconsciousness.

diabetic foods Food products targeted at people with diabetes, in which ordinary sugar (*sucrose*) is replaced with substitutes such as *fructose* or *sorbitol*. These foods are not recommended as part of your food plan.

diabetic nephropathy Type of kidney damage that may occur in diabetes.

diabetic neuropathy Type of nerve damage that may occur in diabetes.

diabetic retinopathy Type of eye disease that may occur in diabetes.

dietary fibre Part of plant material that resists digestion and gives bulk to the diet. Also called fibre or roughage.

diuretics Agents that increase the flow of urine, usually called water tablets.

epidural Usually referring to the type of anaesthetic that is commonly used in obstetrics. Anaesthetic solution is injected through the spinal canal to numb the lower part of the body.

fibre Another name for *dietary fibre*.

fructosamine Measurement of diabetes *control* that reflects the average blood glucose level over the previous 2–3 weeks. Similar to *haemoglobin A$_{1c}$* which averages the blood glucose over the longer period of 2–3 months.

fructose Type of sugar found naturally in fruit and honey. Since it does not require insulin for its *metabolism*, it is often used as a sweetener in *diabetic foods*.

gangrene Death of a part of the body due to a very poor blood supply. A combination of *neuropathy* and *arteriosclerosis* may result in infection of unrecognized injuries to the feet. If neglected this infection may spread, causing further destruction.

gene Unit of heredity controlling a particular inherited characteristic of an individual.

gestational diabetes Diabetes occurring during pregnancy, which recovers at the end of pregnancy.

glargine A new insulin analogue designed to last for 24 hours to act as basal (background) insulin. Also called Lantus.

glaucoma Disease of the eye causing increased pressure inside the eyeball.

glitazones A group of drugs that reduce insulin resistance – see *thiozolidinedione*.

glucagon A *hormone* produced by the *alpha cells* in the *pancreas* which causes a rise in blood glucose by freeing *glycogen* from the liver. Available in injection form for use in treating a severe *hypo*.

glucose Form of sugar made by digestion of *carbohydrates*. Absorbed into the blood stream where it circulates and is used for energy.

glucose tolerance test Test used in the diagnosis of *diabetes mellitus*. The *glucose* in the blood is measured at intervals before and after the person has drunk a large amount of glucose whilst fasting.

glycogen The form in which *carbohydrate* is stored in the liver and muscles. It is often known as animal starch.

glycaemic index (GI) A way of describing how a *carbohydrate*-containing food affects blood *glucose* levels.

glycosuria Presence of *glucose* in the urine.

glycosylated haemoglobin Another name for *haemoglobin A_{1c}*.

haemoglobin A_{1c} The part of the haemoglobin or colouring matter of the red blood cell which has *glucose* attached to it. A test of diabetes *control*. The amount of haemoglobin A_{1c} in the blood depends on the average blood glucose level over the previous 2–3 months.

honeymoon period Time when the dose of insulin drops shortly after starting insulin treatment. It is the result of partial recovery of insulin secretion by the *pancreas*. Usually the honeymoon period only lasts for a few months.

hormone Substance generated in one gland or organ which is carried by the blood to another part of the body to control another organ. *Insulin* and *glucagon* are both hormones.

human insulin Insulin that has been manufactured to be identical to that produced in the human *pancreas*. Differs slightly from older insulins, which were extracted from cows or pigs.

hydramnios An excessive amount of amniotic fluid, i.e. the fluid surrounding the baby before birth.

hyperglycaemia High blood glucose (above 10 mmol/l).

hypo Abbreviation for *hypoglycaemia*.

hypoglycaemia (also known as a hypo or an insulin reaction) Low blood glucose (below 3.5 mmol/l).

impotence Failure of erection of the penis.

injector Device to aid injections.

Innolet A simple injector for insulin designed for people with poor vision or problems with their hands such as arthritis.

insulin A *hormone* produced by the *beta cells* of the *pancreas* and responsible for control of blood glucose. Insulin can only be given by injection because digestive juices destroy its action if taken by mouth.

insulin coma Extreme form of *hypoglycaemia* associated with unconsciousness and sometimes convulsions.

insulin dependent diabetes (abbreviation IDD) Former name for *Type 1 diabetes.*

insulin pen Device that resembles a large fountain pen that takes a cartridge of *insulin*. The injection of insulin is given after dialling the dose and pressing a button that releases the insulin.

insulin reaction Another name for *hypoglycaemia* or a hypo. In America it is called an insulin shock or shock.

insulin resistance A condition where the normal amount of insulin is not able to keep the blood glucose level down to normal. Such people need large doses of insulin to control their diabetes. The glitazone group of tablets is designed to reduce insulin resistance.

intermediate-acting insulin Insulin preparations with action lasting 12–18 hours.

intradermal Meaning 'into the skin'. Usually refers to an injection given into the most superficial layer of the skin. *Insulin* must not be given in this way as it is painful and will not be absorbed properly.

intramuscular A deep injection into the muscle.

islets of Langerhans Specialized cells within the *pancreas* that produce *insulin* and *glucagon*.

isophane A form of *intermediate-acting insulin* that has protamine added to slow its absorption.

joule Unit of work or energy used in the metric system. About 4.18 joules in each calorie. Some dietitians calculate food energy in joules.

juvenile-onset diabetes Outdated name for *Type 1 diabetes*, so called because most patients receiving insulin develop diabetes under the age of 40. The term is no longer used because Type 1 diabetes can occur at any age, although more commonly in young people.

ketoacidosis A serious condition due to lack of insulin which results in body fat being used up to form *ketones* and acids. Characterized by high blood glucose levels, ketones in the urine, vomiting, drowsiness, heavy laboured breathing and a smell of *acetone* on the breath.

ketones Acid substances (including *acetone*) formed when body fat is used up to provide energy.

ketonuria The presence of *acetone* and other *ketones* in the urine. Detected by testing with a special testing stick (Ketostix, Ketur Test). Presence of ketones in the urine is due to lack of *insulin* or periods of starvation.

laser treatment Process in which laser beams are used to treat a damaged *retina* (back of the eye). Used in *photocoagulation*.

lente insulin A form of *intermediate-acting insulin* that has zinc added to slow its absorption.

lipoatrophy Loss of fat from injection sites. It used to occur before the use of highly purified insulins.

lipohypertrophy Fatty swelling usually caused by repeated injections of insulin into the same site.

maturity-onset diabetes Another term for *Type 2 diabetes* most commonly occurring in people who are middle-aged and overweight.

metabolic rate Rate of oxygen consumption by the body, rate at which you 'burn up' the food you eat.

metabolism Process by which the body turns food into energy.

metformin A *biguanide* tablet that works by reducing the release of *glucose* from the liver and increasing the uptake of glucose into the muscle.

microaneurysms Small red dots on the *retina* at the back of the eye which are one of the earliest signs of diabetic *retinopathy*. Represent areas of weakness of the very small blood vessels in the eye. Microaneurysms do not affect the eyesight in any way.

micromole One thousandth (1/1000) of a millimole.

millimole Unit for measuring the concentration of glucose and other substances in the blood. Blood glucose is measured in millimoles per litre (mmol/l). It has replaced milligrammes per decilitre (mg/dl or mg%) as a unit of measurement although this is still used in some other countries. 1 mmol/l = 18 mg/dl.

nateglinide A prandial glucose regulator.

nephropathy Kidney damage. In the first instance this makes the kidney more leaky so that *albumin* appears in the urine. At a later stage it may affect the function of the kidney and in severe cases lead to kidney failure.

neuropathy Damage to the nerves, which may be *peripheral neuropathy* or *autonomic neuropathy*. It can occur with diabetes especially when poorly controlled, but also has other causes.

non-insulin dependent diabetes (abbreviation NIDD) Former name for *Type 2 diabetes*.

orlistat A tablet that blocks the digestion of fat. Brand name Xenical. Used to help people lose weight, which in turn may improve control of diabetes.

pancreas Gland lying behind the stomach, which as well as secreting a digestive fluid (pancreatic juice) also produces the *hormones insulin* and *glucagon*. Contains *islets of Langerhans*.

peripheral neuropathy Damage to the nerves supplying the muscles and skin. This can result in diminished sensation, particularly in the feet and legs, and in muscle weakness. May also cause pain in the feet or legs.

phimosis Inflammation and narrowing of the foreskin of the penis.

photocoagulation Process of treating diabetic *retinopathy* with light beams, either laser beams or xenon arc. This technique focuses a beam of light on a very tiny area of the *retina*. This beam is so intense that it causes a very small burn, which may close off a leaking blood vessel or destroy weak blood vessels that are at risk of bleeding.

pioglitazone A tablet that targets insulin resistance. Trade name Actos.

polydipsia Being excessively thirsty and drinking too much. It is a symptom of untreated diabetes.

polyuria The passing of large quantities of urine due to excess *glucose* from the blood stream. It is a symptom of untreated diabetes.

pork insulin Insulin extracted from the *pancreas* of pigs.

prandial glucose regulators Tablets taken before meals that stimulate the release of *insulin* from the *pancreas* (repaglinide and nateglinide). Only used in *Type 2 diabetes*.

protein One of the classes of food that is necessary for growth and repair of tissues. Found in fish, meat, eggs, milk and pulses. Can also refer to *albumin* when found in the urine.

proteinuria *Protein* or *albumin* in the urine.

pruritus vulvae Irritation of the vulva (the genital area in women). Caused by an infection that occurs because of an excess of sugar in the urine and is often an early sign of diabetes in the older person. It clears up when the blood glucose levels return to normal and the sugar disappears from the urine.

pyelonephritis Inflammation and infection of the kidney.

renal threshold The level of *glucose* in the blood above which it will begin to spill into the urine. The usual renal threshold for glucose in the blood is about 10 mmol/l, i.e. when the blood glucose rises above 10 mmol/l, glucose appears in the urine.

repaglinide A prandial glucose regulator.

retina Light sensitive coat at the back of the eye.

retinopathy Damage to the *retina*.

rosiglitazone A tablet that targets *insulin resistance*. Trade names Avandia and Avandamet (in combination with metformin).

roughage Another name for *dietary fibre*.

saccharin A synthetic sweetener that is *calorie* free.

short-acting insulin Insulin preparations with action lasting 6–8 hours.

Snellen chart Chart showing rows of letters in decreasing sizes. Used for measuring *visual acuity*.

sorbitol A chemical related to sugar and alcohol that is used as a sweetening agent in foods as a substitute for ordinary sugar. It has no significant effect upon the blood *glucose* level but has the same number of *calories* as ordinary sugar so should not be used by those who need to lose weight. Poorly absorbed and may have a laxative effect.

steroids *Hormones* produced by the adrenal glands, testes and ovaries. Also available in synthetic form. Tend to increase the blood *glucose* level and make diabetes worse.

subcutaneous injection An injection beneath the skin into the layer of fat that lies between the skin and muscle. The normal way of giving *insulin*.

sucrose A sugar (containing *glucose* and *fructose* in combination) derived from sugar cane or sugar beet (i.e. ordinary table sugar). It is a pure *carbohydrate*.

sulphonylureas Antidiabetes tablets that lower the blood *glucose* by stimulating the *pancreas* to produce more insulin. Commonly used sulphonylureas are gliclazide and glibenclamide.

thiazolidenedione Generic name for group of tablets that target insulin resistance and improve diabetes in *Type 2 diabetes*. Pharmaceutical names are rosiglitazone and pioglitazone, brand names are Avandia and Actos.

thrombosis Clot forming in a blood vessel.

tissue markers *Proteins* on the outside of cells in the body that are genetically determined.

toxaemia Poisoning of the blood by the absorption of toxins. Usually refers to the toxaemia of pregnancy, which is characterized by high blood pressure, *proteinuria* and ankle swelling.

Type 1 diabetes Name for insulin dependent diabetes which cannot be treated by diet and tablets alone. Outdated name is juvenile-onset diabetes. Age of onset is usually below the age of 40 years.

Type 2 diabetes Name for non-insulin dependent diabetes. Age of onset is usually above the age of 40 years, often in people who are overweight. These people do not always need insulin treatment and usually can be successfully controlled with diet alone or diet and tablets. Formerly known as maturity-onset diabetes.

U40 insulin The old weaker strength of *insulin*, no longer available in the UK. It is still available in Eastern Europe and in some countries in the Far East, such as Vietnam and Indonesia.

U100 insulin The standard strength of *insulin* in the UK, USA, Canada, Australia, New Zealand, South Africa, the Middle East and the Far East.

urine testing The detection of abnormal amounts of *glucose*, *ketones*, *protein* or blood in the urine, usually by means of urine testing sticks.

virus A very small organism capable of causing disease.

viscous fibre A type of *dietary fibre* found in pulses (peas, beans and lentils) and some fruit and vegetables.

visual acuity Acuteness of vision. Measured by reading letters on a sight testing chart (a *Snellen chart*).

water tablets The common name for *diuretics*.

Xenical The brand name for *orlistat*.

Appendix 1
Blood glucose meters

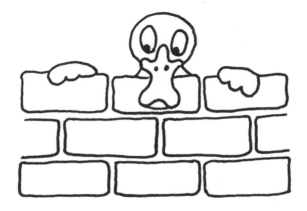

As far as we know, all the information in the table was correct when this book was printed. However, research and changes in technology mean that manufacturers are constantly updating their meters, and the prices also change at frequent intervals. *Balance*, Diabetes UK's magazine, usually carries advertisements for the latest meters. You can check current prices by contacting the manufacturers – their addresses are given in Appendix 3.

Meter	Manufacturer	Type of strip	Time (seconds)
OneTouch Profile	LifeScan	OneTouch test strips	45
OneTouch Ultra	LifeScan	OneTouch Ultra test strips	5
PocketScan	LifeScan	PocketScan test strips	15
AccuChek Advantage	Roche	Advantage 2 test strips	25
AccuChek Active	Roche	Active test strips	5
Ascensia Esprit 2	Bayer	Ascensia GLUCODISC	30
Ascensia BREEZE	Bayer	Ascensia AUTODISC	30
FreeStyle	TheraSense	FreeStyle test strips	15
Supreme Plus	Hypoguard	Hypoguard Supreme	35–60
Precision QID	MediSense	MediSense G2	20
MediSense Optium	MediSense	MediSense Optium	20
Boots Blood Glucose Monitor	Boots	MediSense Optium	20
Soft-Sense can	MediSense	Soft-Sense	20
Prestige Smart System	DiagnoSys Medical	PrestigeSmart System	50
GlucoMen Glyco	A. Menarini Diagnostics	GlucoMen Sensors	30
GlucoMen PC	A. Menarini Diagnostics	GlucoMen Sensors	30

Download to computer	Blood glucose range (mmol/ litre)	Memory (number of results recalled)	Extra features
yes	0–33.3	250 with date and time	can record meals and insulin
yes	1.0–33.3	150 with date and time	can be used for arm testing
yes	1.1–33.3	150 with date and time	very small blood sample required no cleaning necessary
yes	0.6–33.3	100 with date and time	easy to use
yes	0.6–33.3	200 with date and time	very fast test
yes	0.6–33.3	100 with date and time	facility for 4 specific time averages
yes	0.6–33.3	100 with date and time	facility for 4 specific time averages; auto calibration
yes	1.1–27.8	250 with date and time 14-day average	very small blood sample required suitable for arm testing
no	2.0–22.2	70 with date and time	if timed for 60 seconds, can use comparative colour chart
yes	1.1–33.3	10 no date and time	
yes	1.1–44.4	450 with date and time	can also test for blood ketones
yes	1.1–44.4	450 with date and time	very small blood sample required
yes	1.7–25.0	450 with date and time	meter also takes blood sample, be used on arm and base of thumb
no	1.4–33.3	365 no date and time	large clear dispay
no	1.1–33.3	10 no date and time	
yes	1.1–33.3	350 with date and time	strip ejector button

Appendix 2
Useful publications

At the time of writing, all the publications listed here were available. Those available from Diabetes UK (address in Appendix 3) are marked with an asterisk. Check with your local bookshop or Diabetes UK for current prices.

About diabetes

Books

Living with Diabetes*, by Jenny Bryan, published by Hodder Wayland
Diabetes and Your Teenager*, by Bonnie Estridge, published by Thorsons
Late Onset Diabetes*, by Rowan Hillson, published by Vermilion

Magazines and booklets

These titles are all published by Diabetes UK:
Balance* – Diabetes UK's own magazine which appears every other month
Diabetes for Beginners: Type 1*
Diabetes for Beginners: Type 2*
What Diabetes Care to Expect*

Nutrition

Apart from the books listed here, you will also be able to find other titles in your local library. Do check their suitability with your own diabetes clinic before using them, as they may well be out-of-date and include information that is not in line with current dietary recommendations for people with diabetes. The Health Development Agency has useful leaflets for people with diabetes and on healthy eating.

Books and leaflets

The Diabetes Cookbook* by Azmina Govindji and Stella Bowling, published by Sainsbury's in collaboration with Diabetes UK, and available in Sainsbury's supermarkets

The Essential Diabetic Cookbook* by Azmina Govindji and Jill Myers, published by Thorsons in collaboration with Diabetes UK

The Everyday Diabetic Cookbook* by Stella Bowling, published by Grub Street in collaboration with Diabetes UK

Festive Food and Easy Entertaining* by Jill Myers and Azmina Govindji, published by Thorsons in collaboration with Diabetes UK

Food and Diabetes: food choices*, available from Diabetes UK

On Eating, by Susie Orbach, published by Penguin Books

Recipe books

These titles are all published by Diabetes UK:
Home Preserves*
Everyday Cookery* – Healthy recipes for the older person
Home Baking*
Microwave Cookery*
Managing Your Weight*

Appendix 3
Useful addresses

A. Menarini Diagnostics
Wharfedale Road
Winnersh
Wokingham RG41 5RA
Tel: 01189 444 100
Fax: 01189 444 111
Website: www.menarinidiag.co.uk

Aventis Pharma
Aventis House
50 Kings Hill Avenue
Kingshill
West Malling ME19 4AH
Tel: 01732 584000
Fax: 01732 584080
Website: www.aventis.com
Distributor of drugs.

Bayer
Bayer House
Strawberry Hill
Newbury RG14 1JA
Helpline: 01635 566366
Tel: 01635 563000
Fax: 01635 566260
Website: www.bayer.co.uk
Manufactures blood glucose monitoring sytems and meters, and offers advice.

BD
Diabetes Health Care Division
21 Between Towns Road
Cowley OX4 3LY
Tel: 01865 748844
Fax: 01865 717313
Website: www.bddiabetes.com
Manufacture drugs, provide information.

Bio Diagnostics
Upton Industrial Estate
Rectory Road
Upton upon Severn WR8 0LX
Tel: 01684 592262
Fax: 01684 592501
Manufacture medical diagnostic kits.

British Heart Foundation (BHF)
14 Fitzhardinge Street
London W1H 6DH
Helpline: 08450 708070
Tel: 020 7935 0185
Fax: 020 7486 5820
Website: www.bhf.org.uk
Funds research, promotes education & raises money to buy equipment to treat heart disease. For list of publications,

posters and videos, send s.a.e.
Their helpline, HeartstartUK, can
arrange training in emergency
life-saving techniques for lay
people.

British Parachute Association
5 Wharf Way
Glen Parva
Leicester LE2 9TF
Tel: 01162 785271
Fax: 01162 477662
Website: www.bpa.org.uk
Governing body of sport
parachuting. Offers medical
assessment on suitability for
parachuting to people with
medical disorders.

British Sub-Aqua Club
Telfords Quay
Ellesmere Port
Wirral L65 4FY
Tel: 01513 506200
Fax: 01513 506215
Website: www.bsac.com
Governing body for sub-aqua
sport. Offers medical assessment
for those with medical disorders
wanting to take part in diving
underwater.

CP Pharmaceuticals
Ash Road North
Wrexham Industrial Estate
Wrexham LL13 9UF
Tel: 01978 661261
www.cppharma.co.uk

Cygnus UK
First Base, Beacon Tree Plaza
Gillette Way
Reading RG2 0BS
Helpline: 01506 814868
Tel: 01189 319720
Fax: 01189 319721
Website: www.glucowatch.com
Mail order supplier of blood sugar
monitor 'Glucowatch'.

Department of Health (DoH)
PO Box 777
London SE1 6XH
Helpline: 0800 555777
Tel: 020 7210 4850
Fax: 01623 724524
Website:
www.doh.gov.uk/nsf/diabetes.htm
Produces and distributes
literature about public health,
including matters relating to food
allergy. National Service
Framework for Diabetes can be
obtained from internet www.
doh.gov.uk/nsf/diabetes.htm

Diabetes Research and Wellness
Foundation
101–102 North Ney Marina
Hayling Island PO11 0NH
Tel: 02392 637 08
Fax: 02392 636137
Website:
www.diabeteswellnessnet.org.uk
Funds medical research; its
membership receive newsletters
with personal stories and question
and answer section.

Diabetes UK
10 Parkway
London NW1 7AA
Helpline: 020 7424 1030
Tel: 020 7424 1000
Fax: 020 7424 1001
Textline: 020 7424 1888
Website: www.diabetes.org.uk
*Provides advice and information
on diabetes; has local support
groups.*

DiagnoSys Medical
1633 Parkway
Solent Business Park
Fareham PO15 7AH
Helpline: 0800 08 588 08
Tel: 01489 864320
Fax: 01489 864321
*Distributors of blood glucose
monitors and a range of other
products via mail order.*

**Diesetronic Medical
Systems**
The Deer Park Business Centre
Stoneleigh Deer Park
Stareton
Kenilworth CV8 2LY
Tel: 02476 531338
Fax: 02476 531345
Website: www.diesetronic.com
*Manufactures and offers
information about insulin pumps.*

Disability Alliance
First Floor East
Universal House
88–94 Wentworth Street
London E1 7SA
Helpline: 020 7247 8763
Tel: 020 7247 8776
Fax: 020 7247 8765
Website:
www.disabilityalliance.org
*Offers a rights service on social
security benefits. Produces the
Disability Rights Handbook.
Updated three times a year, it
addresses every aspect of social
services benefits for people with
disabilities. Offers advice on
benefits and training for other
organisations and is involved
with policy issues.*

GlaxoSmithKline
Stockley Park West
Uxbridge UB11 1BT
Helpline: 0800 221441
Tel: 020 8990 9000
Fax: 020 8990 4321
Website: www.gsk.com
*Manufacture drugs, provide
information for people via
helpline.*

**The Guide Dogs for the Blind
Association**
Hillfields
Burghfield Common
Reading RG7 3YG
Tel: 0870 600 2323
Fax: 0118 983 5433
Website:
www.guidedogs@gdba.org.uk
*Provides guide dogs, mobility and
other rehabilitation services that*

enable blind and partially sighted people to lead the fullest and most independent lives possible.

Health Development Agency
Trevelyan House
30 Great Peter Street
London SW1P 2HW
Tel: 020 7430 0850
Fax: 020 7413 8900
Website: www.hda-online.org.uk
Formerly Health Education Authority.

Heart UK
7 North Road
Maidenhead SL6 1PE
Tel: 01628 628638
Fax: 01628 628698
Website: www.heartuk.org.uk
Will help anyone at high risk of heart attack, but specializes in inherited conditions causing high cholesterol (ie familial hyper-cholesterolaemia).

HeartstartUK *see under* **British Heart Foundation**

Hypoguard
Dock Lane
Melton
Woodbridge IP12 1PE
Helpline: 0800 371957
Tel: 01394 387333
Fax: 01394 380152
Website: www.hypoguard.com
Distributors of diabetes strips and meters. Involved in research and development.

**The Impotence Association
(now known as The Sexual
Dysfunction Association)**
PO Box 10296
London SW17 9WH
Tel: 020 8767 7791
Fax: 020 8516 7725
Website: www.impotence.org.uk
Offers a listening ear and information on currently prescribed treatment and how sufferers should proceed to get best advice. Can advise on local specialists in erectile dysfunction.

Insulin Dependent Diabetes Trust
PO Box 294
Northampton NN1 4XS
Tel: 01604 622837
Fax: 01604 622838
Website: www.iddtinternational.org
Trust set up to help and advise people having problems with human insulin. Collects insulin for distribution in developing countries. Also runs 'Sponsor a child scheme' for a clinic in India.

Insulin Pump Therapy Group
9 Grafton Gardens
Lymington SO41 8AS
Tel: 01590 677911
Fax: 01590 677763
Website:
www.webshowcase.net/input
Offers information on the use of pumps and puts people in touch with each other. Advises on obtaining funding if pumps are not available via the NHS.

**John Bell & Croyden,
Dispensing Pharmacy**
50–54 Wigmore Street
London W1U 2AU
Tel: 020 7935 5555
Fax: 020 7935 9605
Website:
www.johnbellcroyden.co.uk
*Pharmacy that can obtain
medicines not manufactured in
the UK, with appropriate named
patient prescription and import
licence.*

**Juvenile Diabetes Research
Foundation**
19 Angel Gate
City Road
London EC1V 2PT
Tel: 020 7713 2030
Fax: 020 7713 2031
Website: www.jdrf.org.uk
*Dedicated to funding research to
find a cure for Type 1 diabetes.
Provides information on the
progress of research via leaflets,
newsletters and open meetings.*

LifeScan
Enterprise House
Station Road
Loudwater
High Wycombe HP10 9UF
Helpline: 0800 121200
Tel: 01494 450423
Fax: 01494 463299
Website: www.lifescan.com
*Manufactures blood glucose
monitoring systems and meters.
Offers advice.*

Eli Lilly Diabetes Care Division
Dextra Court
Chapel Hill
Basingstoke RG21 5SY
Helpline: 0800 850777
Tel: 01256 315000
Fax: 01256 315058
Website: www.lilly.com
*Pharmaceutical company. Offers
helpline to people with diabetes.*

Medic-Alert Foundation
1 Bridge Wharf
156 Caledonian Road
London N1 9UU
Helpline: 0800 581420
Tel: 020 7833 3034
Fax: 020 7713 5653
Website: www.medicalert.org.uk
*Offers a body-worn identification
system for people with hidden
medical conditions. Has 24 hour
emergency telephone number.
Offers selection of jewellery with
internationally recognised
medical symbol.*

MediSense Britain
Mallory House
Vanwall Business Park
Maidenhead SL6 4UD
Helpline: 0500 467466
Tel: 01628 773355
Fax: 01628 678808
Order line: 0845 607 3247
Website:
www.abbottlaboratories.com
*Manufactures blood glucose
monitoring systems and meters,
and provides information.*

**The National Institute for
Clinical Excellence**
11 Strand
London WC2N 5HR
Website: www. nice.org.uk

National Kidney Federation
6 Stanley Street
Worksop S81 7HX
Helpline: 0845 601 0209
Tel: 01909 487795
Fax: 01909 481723
Website: www.kidney.org.uk
*Provides information, campaigns
for improvement in care and
supports people through its
network of local groups.*

Novartis
Frimley Business Park
Camberley GU16 7SR
Helpline: 01276 698370
Tel: 01276 692255
Fax: 01276 692508
Website: www.novartis.com
Manufactures drugs.

**Novo Nordisk
Pharmaceuticals**
Broadfield Park
Brighton Road
Crawley RH11 9RT
Helpline: 0845 600 5055
Tel: 01293 613555
Fax: 01293 613535
Website: www.novonordisk.co.uk
*Manufactures injecting pens for
diabetes, growth hormone and
HRT injections.*

Owen Mumford
Brook Hill
Woodstock
Oxford OX20 1TU
Helpline: 0800 731 6959
Tel: 01993 812021
Fax: 01993 813466
Website: www.owenmumford.com
*Manufactures medical products
for diabetics.*

Roche Diagnostics
Diabetes and Point of Care
Rapid Diagnostics
Bell Lane
Lewes BN7 1LG
Helpline: 0800 701000
Tel: 01273 480444
Fax: 01273 480266
Website: www.roche.com
*Manufactures blood glucose
monitoring systems and meters,
and offers advice.*

**The Royal National Institute
of the Blind**
105 Judd Street
London WC1H 9NE
Helpline: 0845 766 9999
Tel: 020 7388 1266
Fax: 020 7388 2034
Website: www.rnib.org.uk
*Offers a range of information and
advice on lifestyle changes and
employment for people facing loss
of sight. Also offers support and
training in braille. Has mail order
catalogue of useful aids.*

Servier Laboratories
Metabolism
Fulmer Hall
Windmill Road
Fulmer
Slough SL3 6HH
Tel: 01753 662744
Fax: 01753 663456
Manufacture diabetes meters,
offer advice.

Stroke Association
Stroke House
123–127 Whitecross Street
London EC1Y 8JJ
Helpline: 0845 303 3100
Tel: 020 7566 0300
Fax: 020 7490 2686
Website: www.stroke.org.uk
Funds research and provides
information now specialising in
stroke only.

Sydney University's Glycaemic
Index Research Service
(SUGiRS)
Human Nutrition Unit
Department of Biochemistry GO8
Sydney University
New South Wales, 2006
Australia
Tel: 0061 2 9351 3757
Fax: 0061 2 9351 6022
Website: www.glycemicindex.com
Commercial research and
advisory service that measures
GI values for foods, drinks and
nuitritional supplements.
Provides advice to manufacturers
to assist them in making low-GI
products.

Takeda Pharmaceuticals
Takeda House
Mercury Park
Wycombe Lane
Wooburn Green
High Wycombe HP10 0HH
Tel: 01628 537900
Fax: 01628 526615
Website: www.takeda.co.uk
Pharmaceutical manufacturers.

Therasense
Centaur House
Ancells Business Park
Ancells Road
Fleet GU51 2UJ
Customer Service line:
0800 138 5467
Tel: 01252 761392
Fax: 01252 761393
Website: www.therasense.com
Manufactures blood glucose
meters.

Tyco Healthcare
154 Fareham Road
Gosport PO13 0AS
Tel: 01329 244226
Fax: 01329 244334
Website: www.tyco.com

Index

Have you found **Diabetes – the 'at your fingertips' guide** practical and useful? If so, you may be interested in other books from Class Publishing.

Type 1 Diabetes in children, adolescents and young adults
Dr Ragnar Hanas £19.99
This practical handbook shows you what you need to take control of your diabetes. It is intended for people with diabetes who are currently using insulin, or planning to do so – an increasing proportion of those with diabetes. Modern research shows unambiguously that a lower mean blood glucose will lessen the risk of late complications. By reading this book you will learn how this can be accomplished easily and fit into your lifestyle.

High Blood Pressure – the 'at your fingertips' guide
THIRD EDITION £14.99
Professor Tom Fahey, Professor Deirdre Murphy and Dr Julian Tudor Hart
The authors use all their years of experience as blood pressure experts to answer over 340 real questions on high blood pressure, including questions you may feel uneasy about asking your doctor, as well as offering positive, practical advice on every aspect of your blood pressure.

'Readable and comprehensive information.'
Dr Sylvia McLaughlan, Former Director General, The Stroke Association

Heart Health – the 'at your fingertips' guide
THIRD EDITION £14.99
Dr Graham Jackson
This practical handbook, written by a leading cardiologist, answers all your questions about heart conditions. It tells you all about you and your heart; how to keep your heart healthy, or if it has been affected by heart disease – how to make it as strong as possible.

'Contains the answers the doctor wishes he had given if only he'd had the time.'
Dr Thomas Stuttaford, The Times

Stop that heart attack!
THIRD EDITION £14.99
Dr Derrick Cutting
The easy, drug-free and medically accurate way to cut your risk of having a heart attack dramatically. Even if you already have heart disease, you can halt and even reverse its progress by following Dr Cutting's simple steps. Don't be a victim – take action NOW!

'This book should be compulsory reading at an early age.'
British Journal of Cardiology

Kidney Dialysis and Transplants – the 'at your fingertips' guide
£14.99
Dr Andy Stein and Janet Wild with Juliet Auer
A practical handbook for anyone with long-term kidney failure or their families. The book contains answers to over 450 real questions actually asked by people with end-stage renal failure, and offers positive, clear and medically accurate advice on every aspect of living with the condition.

'A first class book on kidney dialysis and transplants that is simple and accurate, and can be used to equal advantage by doctors and their patients.'
Dr Thomas Stuttaford, The Times

Beating Depression – the 'at your fingertips' guide
£17.99
Dr Stefan Cembrowicz and Dr Dorcas Kingham
Depression is one of most common illnesses in the world – affecting up to one in four people at some time in their lives. *Beating Depression* shows sufferers and their families that they are not alone, and offers tried and tested techniques for overcoming depression.

'A sympathetic and understanding guide.'
Marjorie Wallace, Chief Executive, SANE

PRIORITY ORDER FORM

Cut out or photocopy this form and send it (post free in the UK) to:

Class Publishing (Priority Service)
FREEPOST 16705
Macmillan Distribution
Basingstoke
RG21 6ZZ

Tel: 01256 302 699
Fax: 01256 812 558

Please send me urgently
(tick boxes below)

Post included
price per copy (UK only)

☐ **Diabetes – the 'at your fingertips' guide** £17.99
(ISBN 1 85959 087 X)

☐ **Type 1 Diabetes in children, adolescents and young adults** £24.99
(ISBN 1 85959 078 0)

☐ **High Blood Pressure – the 'at your fingertips' guide** £17.99
(ISBN 1 85959 090 X)

☐ **Heart Health – the 'at your fingertips' guide** £17.99
(ISBN 1 85959 097 7)

☐ **Sexual Health for Men – the 'at your fingertips' guide** £17.99
(ISBN 1 85959 011 X)

☐ **Stop that heart attack!** £17.99
(ISBN 1 85959 096 9)

☐ **Kidney Dialysis and Transplants – the 'at your fingertips' guide** £17.99
(ISBN 1 85959 046 2)

☐ **Beating Depression – the 'at your fingertips' guide** £20.99
(ISBN 1 85959 063 2)

TOTAL _____

Easy ways to pay

Cheque: I enclose a cheque payable to Class Publishing for £ _____

Credit card: Please debit my   ☐ Mastercard   ☐ Visa   ☐ Switch

Number _____   Expiry date _____

Name _____

My address for delivery is _____

_____

Town _____ County _____ Postcode _____

Telephone number *(in case of query)* _____

Credit card billing address if different from above _____

_____

Town _____ County _____ Postcode _____

Class Publishing's guarantee: remember that if, for any reason, you are not satisfied with these books, we will refund all your money, without any questions asked. Prices and VAT rates may be altered for reasons beyond our control.